W9-ATY-558

To Lucy + Frank
with great
optimism that our
shared dream will
become reality.

Affectionately

Gary Klein

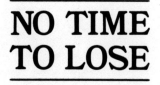

# NO TIME
# TO LOSE

# NO TIME TO LOSE

## GARY KLEIMAN and SANDFORD DODY

WILLIAM MORROW AND COMPANY, INC.

*New York*     *1983*

Copyright © 1983 by Gary Kleiman and Sandford Dody

All rights reserved. No part of this book may be reproduced or utilized in any form or by any means, electronic or mechanical, including photocopying, recording or by any information storage and retrieval system, without permission in writing from the Publisher. Inquiries should be addressed to William Morrow and Company, Inc., 105 Madison Avenue, New York, N.Y. 10016

Library of Congress Cataloging in Publication Data

Kleiman, Gary.
  No time to lose.

    1. Diabetes—Patients—United States—Biography.
2. Kleiman, Gary.   I. Dody, Sandford.   II. Title.
RC660.K58   1983      362.1′96462′00924   [B]      83-707
ISBN 0-688-01822-X

Printed in the United States of America


    2   3   4   5   6   7   8   9   10

BOOK DESIGN BY BERNARD SCHLEIFER

To my mother, my father and my brother—
the best part of my team.

For the remarkable Kleimans—
my new family.
SANDY DODY

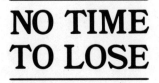

# NO TIME
# TO LOSE

# 1

I GUESS I'm lucky. I was born tough and in a hurry, so I've got a lot done at the age of twenty-eight. I wasn't given the luxury of time, so dawdling has been out of the question—especially now.

Unlike most people, I've never been able to watch idly as the present slips like a thief into the past and then to gaze into a future guaranteed by design. I've had to seize each moment and treasure it, like the gem it is. In consequence, I've lived richly. In a way I can be envied. My greed for life has served me well, although I haven't always been allowed to smell the flowers along the way.

I've had diabetes since I was six and at eighteen I rushed headlong into middle age. At this writing I am medically an old man. It's really bizarre, like Buckminster Fuller being power forward for the Knicks or Methuselah playing with himself and picking at his acne.

Legally blind for the last ten years, only one tiny patch of vision in my left eye, two corroded kidneys, hypertension, vulnerability to a hundred diseases and most irritating of all, a rapidly receding hairline, I found that the business of staying alive which for years was a serious hobby was becoming a fulltime career. The tightrope necessary to negotiate between the extremes of coma and somogyi—which is the reactive excess of insulin and then glucose in the blood—takes the calculations of an Einstein and the fleet grace of a Baryshnikov.

This balance of insulin and glucose must, at all times, be secured and with it a determination of physical activity and, yes, emotional intensity. When for whatever reason, hypoglycemia or low blood sugar is untreated, the body too zealously can compensate thereby creating hyperglycemia, or high blood sugar.

In between the endless shots and calibrations and remedial snacks we who have diabetes must crowd these productive activities that usually enrich and govern the unafflicted person's life. We're kept pretty busy stealing that residual time so many take for granted.

There is no disease on record that makes such constant, minute-to-minute and long-term demands on its victims.

Diabetes mellitus is *incurable*. There is no corrective surgery. There is no remission. It goes its relentless way, and until the people in research find the answers, the stricken must either deny the facts while indulging themselves in fantasy and Baskin-Robbins or try to beat the odds by running as fast as possible to stay in the same place. There is, at least, a slim chance that way. Certainly early control encouraged and mastered in childhood may delay the wicked complications of this unsweetest of diseases. And so I write this book.

For the time being, I'm flat on my ass hooked up to a million wires and tubes. Mr. Machine. I look like something out of *Star Wars*. This should be just for a short time, and while I progress with my story, I will probably become more mobile. But while I'm out of commission, trusting that this is the beginning of a convalescence, I must use the time profitably. This is exactly the right moment to start the book I've been planning to write for years.

Apart from the ego trip which will afford me my first holiday from the unpleasant grind, I must warn the kids I work with and all the others who make up the terrible statistics of juvenile diabetes, that without self-approval and religious control of their disease they could have me to look forward to. The story of my past might just give them a better future. They mustn't go through this. What a fate, being a Boogeyman to children. But if I can convince their parents that there's hope along with discipline and hard work, OK.

I fought control all my life and brother look at me now. And I didn't do it alone. The medical profession was an all too willing collaborator. Not that certain doctors meant me harm. They didn't know any better back in 1960. And not that perfect command over my state of health could have reversed the disease. But it could possibly have delayed for years the crippling complications that can inevitably result from diabetes.

Jesus, how I fought control. All my life. I mean over my sovereignty, my independence, over *me*. I was a monster from the beginning. Rebellious, mischievous, unmanageable. I drove my parents to despair and laughter. Cunning and not without charm, I was a showoff and precocious to the point of inviting strangulation. My energy and the creative use of it for naughtiness, disobedience and flight were to be used less destructively as I grew old.

I certainly didn't choose this murderous game, but I was given the temperament to play it. And to win at all costs. It's interesting. It's almost as if there was a God or Something, because I always felt special and I have detected, I think, a faint attempt at divine justice. I mean, I did come into this world equipped for battle: feisty, hard-assed, determined and outrageous, with helmet and knee guards in place. And I watched myself take charge, virtually usurp control, fighting first for my destiny—and then more decidedly against it.

Nature understands. The porcupine, the turtle, the rose. It isn't that I think there's nothing, absolutely nothing beyond the struggle for survival. My family, my friends are the greatest. There's so much sweetness and laughter, and things are so pretty. Life can be really nice, really great, even if it is a pain in the ass. Now, about God! I don't *not* believe. But I can't honestly say that I feel that anything very serious is going on up there.

The porcupine makes sense, and I have my own shell and thorns. But I work with diabetic children, and when I watch their

*11*

bewildered faces as I teach them how to test their urine with a bright little color chart or show them how, safely, to prick their fingers for that drop of blood that will help better determine their sugar content, I just can't believe somebody planned it this way. I mean, kids toying with their pee and their blood. Right? It's not right.

It makes me angry because I know that never in their whole lives will these kids ever be graced with spontaneity. They will never be able to obey an impulse without a structure system that by its very nature, drains the delayed moment of real pleasure. These kids, some of them four and five, can't be carefree puppies. But, damnit, they'll develop the character of thoroughbreds or languish for its lack.

Diabetic children grow up fast. They develop a sense of responsibility or else. I am determined more than ever that they know that they are not alone, that their burden is noted and most of all, that they have the privilege of enhancing as well as lengthening their lives. That early devotion to their cause can reward them with a possible respite of years that may succeed the Cure for which so many remarkable men and women are now working. The kids must not only grow up but prevail.

As a child I wasn't told how seriously ill I was. My parents were not told. The doctors didn't know. "You should be glad he has diabetes. When he grows up, the army will never take him." "Insulin has saved him." "There doesn't have to be a cure as long as there's insulin." "He'll lead a completely normal life."

All of it—bullshit! My parents and eventually I, as well, were beguiled by all this well-meaning garbage. And we invested the doctors with all manner of wisdom and authority. Actually, for quite some time, I was spared the terrible dividends that were so mercilessly accruing.

Except for my daily shots of insulin and the frequent and clumsy urine testing, despite the prohibition of all the poisoned junk food our nation relishes and ostensibly thrives on, I would seem to have had a really neat childhood—on the face of it. I had immense energy and enthusiasm and all the extra sweets my condition or vivid imagination demanded. I was treated by my parents like a VIP. I mean, really very special, VSOP! Like the best Courvoisier. My brathood, however, was not accepted wholeheartedly and my punishments were as frequent as my parents' solicitude. I drove them to distraction, but my mother and father have a sense of fun that allowed, despite their fury and impatience with my attempted anarchy, for almost continuous laughter. We have always delighted in each other, and the general glow that radiated from our house prepared me greatly to face the darker days to come.

I really thought I was hilarious. I was hyper beyond the beyond and the cross my parents bore. I trust I gave them small pleasures. There is evidence that I did, though it was my brother who was honey while I was brine. I always agitated. Glenn soothed. Aside from my genetic setup—I was born a leading man—*diabetes had made me a superstar* and I liked that part of it—the twinkling bit. I was always on, and that's tough for others to live with. I dissembled and manipulated. I bamboozled the whole family.

Chronically sick people can, of course, tyrannize a household, much as an infant does. That I did so with some dash doesn't alter the fact. I drove everyone wild, and my punishments, though frequent, were to no avail. We will never know how much of my hyperactivity was physiological. I suspect—being privy to some inside information—that some of my satanic behavior I managed with little or no pancreatic assistance. I wasn't born, I exploded. Of course, for the record, there might have been an imbalance before the disease surfaced.

How does a smart little boy who wants his way, has been made to feel different and special, whose energy is irrepressible, know how far he can go? And how far can he be allowed to go without a straitjacket? I was smart and adaptable. It was easy to get my own way since all my victims had a built-in fear factor. Clowning, cavorting with the whole family on that high wire, how could we not be in danger of losing much more than our bal-

13

ance? And I forced the whole gang into the act. The Flying Kleimans. Watch them in their death-defying, laugh-provoking, side-splitting, thrill-a-minute human pyramid, and *without a net*, ladies and gentlemen. And guess who's at the apex. The star attraction. One guess.

# 2

A GUY in my position can't plan ahead with any real assurance. My cause and its effect are pretty much a thing of the past. I should have been wise when I was six years old. I wasn't. Today, I'm forced to live each day as if it had no relation to the preceding or following one. Consciously surviving. That the days have added up and made a mosaic I can discern and describe is not luck or even art by accident. My need to control has magnetized and pulled things into place. My need to be in control created mischief and mayhem when I was small, but when I at last grew up helped create order. I put my best foot forward now, but I never know when the devil will take my hindmost. I've come, perhaps superstitiously, to prepare for the worst and relish the unexpected. I guess I can be called a cockeyed pessimist.

Up to this moment I've moved fast—on the tennis and basketball courts and in and out of the shadows. Partly nervous energy, and mostly because speed is essential. I've done a lot of high stepping, perhaps, in hopes that a swiftly moving target better eludes the hunter. Yup! I've been sort of hung up on death these last years, and certainly in recent weeks. We all try to keep well ahead of the enemy, but most people don't recognize him. We've met, glared each other down and chosen our weapons. Now all the son of a bitch has to do is catch me.

Living with this intelligence is what has made me special. What a way to be special. Who the hell wants to know the end of the story before you're really into it? Hollywood has begged audiences "not to reveal the end of this picture." Well, who the hell is considerate anymore? But I have every intention of doing a rewrite job. Even as I lie here, flat on my back, I'm alert to every step in the hall, every creak of the door and every beat of my pulse. Years ago, when I first became aware of my heartbeat, I heard a drumroll that beckoned me to battle. I might have been an unwilling draftee, but no gung-ho asshole has ever fought so long and fanatically in a war he didn't declare.

Operation operation loomed for years. It was only a matter of time before what we call the numbers game—those blood and urine counts—would add up to surgery, no longer elective but indispensable. The suspense had grown over the years, and then it was unbearable.

My story has enough suspense for a hundred thrillers, and I wish for once in my life I could have the chance of being bored. To live an uneventful life. Well, this was not the script prepared for me and, to tell the truth, I'd probably hate it. On again, off again. They call me the human yo-yo. But this is the worst yet. I who love to play the field, roam the world, be free above all else am on a pretty short leash. For how long, I don't know. It could be forever, and we don't know how long that will be either. I'll keep you posted.

By the time I get on with this, I'm sure I'll be OK. I have to be. I'm programmed to be so fucking noble and brave that I can't disappoint anybody—especially the kids. Lying here—isolated— the reverse of a pariah, unable to be visited by anyone who isn't masked and fumigated, the telephone and tape my only lines of communication, a rush of panic makes me pick up the phone.

One of my kids, a patient at the clinic where I am a counselor, is nine years old. He's already had a couple of errant fathers and his mother—in order to redesign her own life-style—has recently left the city, leaving him with a grandparent. As his counselor, I have been the only constant in his life. Now I have seemingly abandoned him too. I've got to get better fast, and Roger must know that *this* needn't happen to him, that in any case I am here for him to speak to and that, doubtless, I'll be home in a matter of pages and possibly back at work in a couple of chapters.

Has anyone written a book like this? I think it's great, because I've never started anything I didn't finish. That is a fact and immutable. 'Nuff said.

I have come late and reluctantly to humility. As with my sensitivity to medication, I can tolerate only small doses. Still, in quieter, saner moments, I warm to the love and support I've received from family, friends and my present physicians. My story must be theirs. People have always been most important to me. Perhaps because of my history—too important. Nothing in this world gives me more pleasure than sharing. And that is a sometime dissatisfaction, that prime need for interrelationships. It has sabotaged my work as a sculptor.

I love my work. The clay, the marble, the metal, the tools, the smell, the dust. I love it as I used to love drawing and painting; but I love people more. I find it lonely working alone. I have to bounce off people, you know? While working, the artist, sculptor, writer must be monastic, and I ain't no monk. I must always be part of the action, part of a team. Even when my vision and energy level allowed me to play tournament tennis, I loved doubles, a partner that made for dual effort and a relationship—not just an adversary to be beaten.

Some fields allow for joint creativity. Gilbert and Sullivan, Beaumont and Fletcher, the Albrecht and Marx brothers. What a ball being a Marx brother. To make people laugh and never have to be alone. They probably hated each other or something, but the greater reality binds them together forever.

Isamu Noguchi, the sculptor, gave me a set of carving tools that I treasure as much as his genius. He has always been a hero, but years ago he let me down by confessing that not only was "work the only proof that you've been here" but that he had "lost all interest in people." I was really thrown by this, but, of course, it is this inevitable refinement of his work, the ultimate abstraction, that dehumanizes as it soars. Such apotheosis transcends art and trespasses on physics, the impersonality of science.

I guess I'm incapable of such detachment. It can be bloodless. I've got to rub elbows and noses with the rest of the gang, though, frankly, only by my choice. Now really isolated by necessity, I again want to be out there with everybody, and writing this may enable me to do so. It seems that no matter my sometime commitment to art, living is my favorite medium. But, for me, it is a tough one.

No other gratification I've known has equaled that of working with young people and their parents who, I trust, will read this book and learn the easy way. They must neither tyrannize nor coddle. They mustn't spoil the child for survival. And, like one of my latest patients' mothers, they must under no condition go into a panic that must automatically be shared by the patient. Frenzy is contagious. They must, as quickly and as coolly as possible, have the child, no matter what age, share in his own management, because it will be forever. And he must learn fast.

For the diabetic kids everywhere who play my old game of ignoring or falsifying their daily reports, I beg them to get it together. By not testing, they believe they cannot fail. That denial of the disease will erase it. No way. No news is not good news with diabetes. It won't go away. One must learn to live with it equably.

While qualified men and women study and reconstitute the smoking vials in laboratories, we diabetics must cooperate and keep ourselves in shape so we will be ready for the moment of deliverance. It will come, the cure. I know what my parents have done in the cause of diabetic research. Because of me they have, with other engaged families, raised millions of dollars in southern Florida. The answer is in the laboratories, but we who suffer must not be in such a state of disrepair that it will come too late.

Some patients have decided that it is hopeless, that, at best, control is just treading water. That's like telling a swimmer without further endurance that since he can't reach land he should

18

sink. As long as he stays afloat, anything is possible. I believe in miracles. I've seen them. A boat, a helicopter, a goddamned dolphin can come along, but you've got to be there ready for them.

I've seen adolescents, still apparently healthy, either laugh away their reality or with teen-age passion actually embrace it, yielding to the disease like a kind of frustrated virgin. Feast or famine. First I was told that I was lucky to have the damned disease and then I was told that I wouldn't live to be twenty. I've become inured to anything.

The day before I was operated on, my brother, Glenn, called from Connecticut. He and his wife, Gise, which rhymes with Lizzie, were flying down to Miami, were on their way. The family meets everything together and head on.

"Are you nervous, Gar?"

"Well, no. Not yet."

"What the hell are you waiting for?"

My family. I got my genes from them, my A positive blood, my A positive outlook, probably a predisposition to my diabetes and surely my zest for life. After all, where would I be without them?

Lying here, I'm bombarded with memories. Most vividly, I recall my first time in a hospital. It's like a dissolve in a movie. I'm six years old and paralyzed with fear, fighting for my life— and what an adversary.

She was coming at me, my own mother, Marge, with a syringe and a needle half my size and she was more frightened than I. She was convinced that she was going to harm me in this her first attempt to shoot me with the necessary insulin. And I agreed with her. Of course, she wasn't admitting to these terrible reservations, but I saw right through her. I wasn't stupid.

For days, Marge had practiced with oranges, gaily piercing their bright cratered skins and then inserting so many units of water underneath them. I watched her until she became really deft. Now the needle was sterilized and she had graduated to a human being—me. My mother came toward me trembling and smiling in an effort to make me think this was playtime. She was half-crazed and I caught her terror and started screaming. I hid under the covers and then, realizing that I would be trapped there, I kicked her in the chest with all my might and then jumped out of bed. In the next bed I met the frightened eyes of a hemophiliac who imagined that, like many an innocent bystander before him, he would possibly end up the unwitting victim in a bloody spectacle. As he recoiled, I slid under the glass night table of the guy opposite me—a weight lifter—who was spared the drama because he was in a diabetic coma.

While Marge stood her ground, shaking but game, eager to convince us both that she had mastered the now-necessary ritual, a nurse and orderly pulled me across the floor kicking and screaming. The nurse was unreal. She was out of Dickens. "See this poor man?" she asked, nodding toward the unconscious muscleman. "That's what's going to happen to you if you don't watch out." It took four people to hold me down while my mother passed the test with flying colors and then almost passed out herself.

# 3

WE HAD BEEN building "that was a house" to which touchstone all other future homes would have to be unfavorably compared, when I started to wet my bed. Since I'd been born housebroken, this was not only embarrassing but weird. I was considered so uninhibited that Dr. Nina Ellenbogen suggested a possible bladder infection, and then at St. Francis Hospital I was diagnosed as diabetic, and that was Day One. Now, twenty-two years later, I was at County Hospital at Jackson Memorial for two weeks of examinations and instruction.

Marge, of course, became an expert in no time. Anything she does she does perfectly, and for the next few years, she plied her new trade faultlessly. My father, Marty, marveled at her bravery. He couldn't touch me, and the only friction I ever remember between my parents was caused by his inability to substitute for her when my mother had the flu and couldn't minister to me. Neither could he. Not as inner directed, more rhapsodic than my mother, Marty is so giving, open and willing that he'll take a stab at anything except his sons. I remember his holding the syringe and making little, darting motions—vamping until ready, hoping that lightning or earthquake would strike, making the shot unnecessary—until, I guess, my mother *had* to take over or I'd still be waiting.

At nine, I learned to inject myself and learned, literally, at my

21

father's knee. When I finished practicing on oranges, he let me practice on him. I kept tatooing his thigh and his arm until he looked like a junkie. I could do anything to him. I kept jabbing him, sometimes deep into his flesh, until I got it right. He could have been a dart board. And he couldn't touch me once. He's a real softy, my father.

My mother is not. She is the most beautiful, feminine, devoted, dependable and loving Marine drill sergeant in service. She has heard her orders from the top command and nothing will stop her from carrying them out. She also spots a phony before he knocks on the door. I swear, the woman is uncanny—maybe a witch. And this is good because my father, with his infinite goodwill and sunny nature, has to be bound, gagged and robbed before he believes he's in the presence of someone without his best interests at heart.

All I know is that they are a great combination. My mother had always, from my birth, had a tough time controlling me, but after this confrontation she zeroed in and circled me like a hawk. Between scoldings and worse, she became a genius at "needling" me. Her disarming, disobedient brat had become her diabetic and possibly self-destructive child. She became both my fortress and my prison. Her love and concern drove me bananas.

I was always fleeing, always on the run. If she picked me up to cuddle, I wriggled out of her arms and scooted. I couldn't be contained for a moment on laps, in arms or in the house itself. My timing was always great. When I was indoors with a cold or whatever, I plotted and planned, waiting for the exact moment Marge—with an armful of clothes—was at the washing machine. Exquisitely timed, as she would reach for the lever I would bolt and soon be a block away.

Far worse than the classically dreaded "Where are you going?" or "What were you doing?" was the constant "Have you tested, Gary?" I can still hear her demanding an answer. "Have you *tested*, Gary?" It drove me up the wall, partly because I hadn't and also because she was an unwelcome reminder of the illness I wanted to deny. The doctors had been sanguine about my future. Insulin was saving my life and there was never a problem about my responsibilities in that department. I clearly remembered the muscleman. I knew early on that, if I tried to fly out of the upstairs window, I could kill myself. I also knew that not taking insulin could do the same. I wouldn't fly out of windows and I wouldn't not take insulin. But once that was established, what was the big deal? This testing business was a bore, a chore and, more distressingly, a label, a sign that I was different from others—something I didn't come to prefer until later. Still, my mother was after me. "Have you tested, Gary?" She was so rigid that I wanted to oil her like the Tin Man in the *Wizard of Oz*. What the hell did she want from me?

And yet, it was my mother alone who said, "I know he's active and properly naughty, but how can they say he's leading a normal life when every single day he has to shoot all that junk into his little body?"

The woman always cuts through the garbage. But impossible. She is a perfectionist and must always be in control, deferring only to my father when she knows he's right. "Have you tested?" was her favorite of many demanding questions whose answers I would avoid by fleeing. She is compulsive and a CIA filing cabinet. She forgets nothing and everything is in place. I was the one loose end that eluded her, the one thing she could never find when she looked for it. The smirking joker in the pack of cards she had so neatly pigeonholed.

First as a healthy imp and then as a diabetic recalcitrant who rebelled against her intensive care, I remained one step ahead of her, challenging and taunting and spiteful. If she relaxed her vigil for five minutes, I was up to no good. And still, when I was in the mood, I could be loving and even helpful around the house.

At an Easter party in the hospital the first week of my diabetes, I thought I was being a model son and a nice boy when I asked, "Mom, would you like some of these pretty jelly beans?"

While I popped some red and green ones down my throat, Marge almost swooned. It could have been arsenic I was enjoying. And she was right. This candy could have thrown me all out of whack.

"Jelly beans?" she gasped as she tried to empty my fist and

busy mouth while she contemplated a prodding finger or stomach pump.

"Gary! How could you? You know—"

I knew. I had forgotten. I had wanted to forget. I hadn't as yet acknowledged the endless prohibitions that were to restrict and change my life. The jelly-bean incident was innocent; but I could be such a shit.

Not allowed to cross the road in front of our apartment house, I crawled under a water bridge at the end of the street instead. When my mother emerged from the house I called sweetly from across the heavily trafficked road, knowing that she'd look really foolish when I revealed that I really hadn't disobeyed at all. I'd show her. Of course only a water rat and I could have negotiated the narrow seawall along which I'd crawled. She would have far preferred my bucking ten ton trucks.

If diabetes was taking a long time to get me, it's a wonder my mother didn't kill me first.

There was no way I would ever stop challenging her authority. As I grew older, I was sure my mother would prevent me from growing hair on my chest. There were plenty of my victims who would have sworn I sported it on the palms of my hands.

Had I been an adult, I might have understood her devotion and the penalty for rejecting it. But I was a cyclone, not a child, and I couldn't be tempered.

Originally from Manhattan, with a background similar to Lauren Bacall's, Marge—a dyed-in-the-wool New Yorker, still displaced in Florida—also wanted to be an actress. She has managed it. In all stages of her careers as wife, mother and Foundation worker, she has succeeded. There is always drama when Marge is performing. Just as there is always comedy with Marty. From our small apartment to "that was a house" to their present home, my mother has always created handsome settings for our repertory company. She's got style.

Marge will deny this—as Marty denies his faulty hearing—but her love of cleanliness, her demand for the immaculate, led her to dress my brother and me entirely in white for a few years so

24

that she could more readily spot a spot. It was insane. Bizarre. We looked like an Ingmar Bergman flashback and wanted only for silver birches instead of royal palms.

And straitlaced? I must have been about fourteen and Glenn eleven when one day our mother came home fuming. A friend had unexpectedly returned to her home to find her son in her bedroom with a girl. They were red-faced and she caught them red-handed, if I may be anatomically inexact. My mother shared her friend's trauma. "In her own bed!" she kept repeating in shock. The location seemed to distress her more than the act. She now drew us close and delivered an ultimatum. If ever she were to catch either one of us in *her* bed with a girl, it would be the *end*. Such an outrage would result in damnation beyond our nightmares of hell.

Glenn and I were dumbfounded by her outburst. In the first place, at fourteen my hyperactivity had not as yet been concentrated and directed into a sexual drive. I was such an innocent jock that, if I thought of sex at all, it was a mystery not yet unraveled. Still, I was the wise guy who knew all the answers, and Marge had this mad vision of coming home and finding me in *her* bed with Marilyn Monroe. She kept lashing out at me to discourage this plan, which she flatteringly thought I could realize, and then she turned to Glenn—so serious and shy.

"And that goes for you, too, young feller," our mother warned, her eyes blazing.

"But, Mom," Glenn said, "I haven't even reached puberty yet."

My brother not only made family history that day but his sober, honest, sensible response broke the spell, and Marge looked at Glenn and then at me and burst out laughing. In a moment, the *three* of us were rolling on *her* bed gasping with laughter—I mean, but really convulsed.

There has always been, despite everything, laughter in our house. And always talk, no matter how insane. Little goes unsaid. Everything has always been discussed by all four of us, and in a real crisis, Marge and Marty are always a united front. There could never be the possibility of playing one off against the other. I tried.

Early on, I made my mother the target for my pint-sized rage. My meanness seemed to know no horizon. I wanted to get a rise out of her and did. We both wanted to be in charge and the ensuing one hundred years' war was inevitable. But I fought dirty and my mother never did. I used sickness and pity as well as knavery. If all else failed, I'd develop "symptoms." I was the boy who cried "Dr. Wolf."

On one particular day, I was so insufferable to my mother that Marty was forced, as he occasionally was, to punish me. He had only spanked me once, when I was five, but now—years later—he left a far greater mark on me. His very blue eyes nailed me to the spot and there was not a trace of laughter in them.

He said the most unbelievable thing and he said it with terrible calm.

"I do not like the way you're treating my wife!"

That's what he said. Wow! Did I ever get the message.

No, we did not have a good relationship, my mother and I. And my natural orneriness was not sweetened by my sugar. I was both obnoxious and "delicate," a winning combination. I couldn't lose and took advantage of everybody. Though as a child I mostly enjoyed a feeling of well-being, I knew that diabetes mellitus was not a cause for celebration.

It secretly nagged me that, despite all the pie in the sky about my future, my grandmother was not to be told of my illness. My father's mother had had a stroke, and I was informed that, when I visited her and watched her polishing her silver as therapy, I was never to mention diabetes. One more strain or shock, I inferred, might be fatal. It didn't occur to anyone that this warning caged my own fugitive fears and never totally disappeared from my consciousness.

I was much too young to entertain thoughts of mortality, but I was cunning enough to know a perfect weapon when I saw one. And I eventually used it on everyone: like a butter knife on my father, a stiletto on my teachers and other condescending creatures, and as a machete on my mother. It is a wonder that I wasn't tarred and feathered by the Dade County vigilantes led by my own family.

Still, my gusto could be contagious and my tightrope took me many places as I balanced it all with laughter. Just as I was about to go that one step too far, I'd turn on the charm and become so sweet, helpful and affectionate that I disarmed them all. That, ladies and gentlemen, is how to get away with murder and suicide.

I always loved making people laugh and even now—especially now—any wit I can muster and all of my self-deprecating humor allow me better control over the social situations the healthy are ill-equipped to handle. Most people don't know how to act with the seriously sick. I know how tough it is to achieve the perfect balance, but often real compassion prompts one to a pity that verges on contempt. And so I set the tone.

"Look, buddy, you've had a couple. Maybe I should drive." One tries.

From childhood I was made to feel different. I think that really sick people are a mystery that frightens healthy children, making them wary and defensive. My school days were often painful. The morbid curiosity of strangers and the shy solicitude of intimates, the whole kid-gloved approach that indulged me unduly, set me apart where I gladly remained, playing it both ways, inviting gains and losses.

Blithely missing classes, demanding larger desserts, longer rest periods and less responsibility, I both resented my impositions while exploiting diabetes shamelessly. Then there was my height. I was short for so long. I never became a Globetrotter but, at least, I'm up there with the rest of you now—almost.

What a wild one I was, fragmented, sparking, fizzling, raining on everyone like fireworks, and every day I made sure was Independence Day. I was always celebrating.

Don't take your eyes off your little sugar baby. You'll laugh till you cry.

# 4

**M**Y CREATININE is higher and my Blood Urea Nitrogen count affectionately called BUN is puzzlingly astronomical. I hope you're impressed. The doctors aren't sure what it all means but it ain't good. I'm in numbsville. How long can you be depressed?

I just called Marty at his factory.

"Hello, Dad? I just wanted you to know that if you have any Kleiman BUN, sell!"

Marty's my best audience. My father laughs and cries easily. He's really an innocent. And so I take the serious things he says seriously. It's straight from the shoulder. I mean, he knows what he's talking about. You can't miss it. It's in the eyes, the smile, the way he touches you.

His candor, the rest of the family knows, has a price. I don't know how he made it in business. My mother, Glenn and I have explained that the world is filled with villains and he smiles patiently. His trust can disarm hoods and saints, but we fear for him. Though he manages to be a businessman, teacher, father, husband, fund raiser and athlete, he is happily free of the natural suspicions that he would call paranoia. He's like a clear day, my father, and generous as all outdoors.

Intelligent and—despite those hot denials—slightly deaf, he is, I tell you, absolutely blind to the wickedness abroad. I am convinced he would give an unsuccessful mugger a second chance. He seems, however, to be immune to harm, perhaps even charmed. Marge insists that the family couldn't have survived without him. He's as dependable as the unexpected. He is our sounding board, and I've got to hand it to my mother. She knows quality. He in turn is so sure of himself that he recognizes my mother's mysterious connection with the source. It's an unbelievable marriage, and my greatest regret is that I can never have one like it.

Marty's father was "in cheese" and so was he for a while when he graduated from Syracuse University. He had anticipated Sara Lee and tried freezing cheesecake and waffles without the fictitious lady's enormous success. May Rich was the unprophetic name of his product. Newly married, and then, with my arrival, as a brand-new father, Marty set forth with his little family to Florida and what he hoped would be a sunny future. He was a traveling salesman, selling paint and plastics.

After researching modern plastics, he started making little things like acrylic door numbers and then moved on to wall and furniture coverings, vinyl handbags and imitation leather luggage. From selling, he turned to manufacturing, and, with his own formula, made and marketed pool paint to the new rich, some of whom were glad to have had bathtubs up north. It was a different Miami in those days, quiet, only recently settled.

Marty worked twelve hours a day, six days a week, mixing the paint himself. We lived in a small apartment and every night my father would come home looking like a Jackson Pollock canvas. My earliest memories of him were paint-splattered. While Marge would tend to my baby brother, born three years after I was, my father would read the comics to me and make me model airplanes. I remember sitting in his lap picking the dried flecks of paint off him as he fell asleep watching *Perry Mason*. I would pick away like a dedicated ape grooming her young. It's a warming memory. The world was small and safe and easy to tidy up in those days.

Marty's eyes are usually crinkled with laughter. He can sell anything to anybody, but gives himself unreservedly to his family first and then to everybody else. His great success can only be considered a miracle. But, then, I've already said it. He's charmed. And charming. He still, after all our tutoring, will manage to find some redeeming quality in Jack the Ripper or Attila the Hun. It's unbelievable that he has survived, much less done so well for all of us. He's ridiculous and we love him.

In case I've made my father sound like some kind of retarded person, I must make it clear that my mother, who is God's sister-in-law, would be lost without his strength, his understanding and his wisdom. He's the linchpin of the family. It's just that Marty sees the rest of us as a reflection of himself—and if only that were true. He looks at the world through those baby blues and everything is neat, which is really bizarre because *he's* not blind.

And yet, he's either deaf or distracted. For example, Marge, being traditionally Sunday-football-television-casual about supper, said, "How would you like to order some pizza?"

Marty Kleiman—in our presence, I swear to you—answered, "Who's Howard Oates?"

On my life! Marge, Glenn and I were on the floor, I mean on the floor, crying with laughter. "Who's Howard Oates?" this man asked, and I'll tell you. We've decided he's an unsuccessful CPA with six daughters and a nagging wife and every April fifteenth he gets shingles. Howard, we salute you. In our family he has become our hero. We had T-shirts made with his name emblazoned on them. All four of us wore them for years—I guess on his birthday. Anyway, that's my Dad, who is so out of this world sometimes that we call him Morty Kleinberg, which is nearer than he got with Mr. Oates.

Now, for my brother. I know that nobody is going to believe this, but my brother, Glenn, was born in a three-piece suit. He was respectable from the start. The vest was there to conceal an inverted navel, which always fascinated me. I tried for many months to reverse it by poking my finger in it. Everybody objected except Glenn. He loved it.

The day I was told he was born, I dashed out of the house, got on my tricycle and announced his birth up and down the street. Throwing pebbles at windows and doors, I screeched, "I have a baby sister. I have a baby sister."

When I was informed later that a boy was a brother, I repeated the whole business, this time getting it right but cracking a window.

"I have a baby brother!"

How I loved him. I would stand like a dumb animal in a crèche, staring at him in wonder. And I would poke him in that belly button. Glenn would smile a shadow of a smile that I was told was gas but which was the same shadow of a smile he has today.

Glenn thought a lot as a baby and seemed to be reflecting on past memories, which was doubtful because he'd just got here and even if there *is* something before, I think we leave the old wardrobe behind and don't arrive with a set of luggage.

It would be too pat to report that Glenn developed asthma as an attention getter in a house dominated by diabetes and Dionysius, but 'tain't so. He had asthma as an infant, before I became ill and a superstar. My earliest memories have to do with my father improvising a tent over Glenn's crib—a kind of vaporizing affair to stop the terrible wheezing and choking which had my mother and father in a panic. If asthma is, as some say, psychologically induced I don't know what the kid's problem could have been. He was adored by all of us. He might, I suppose, have brought it along in a shoulder bag. I tell you, as an infant, he sat mulling things over.

He was a good baby but after a while, Marge and Marty decided that he was retarded because he wouldn't talk. When the proper time came for a baby to speak he just didn't. That is, he made sounds but not the imitative sounds that slowly approximate the language that surrounds a child. There was not the slightest relationship between his grunts and chirping and any known language.

"Alaraniamilootoona," Glenn would fretfully intone and my

31

mother would put her hands to her mouth in muted grief. She had apparently spawned an idiot.

"Perhaps if we looked it up," Marty would volunteer but my mother saw no humor in the situation.

"You see, Gary, how important it is to speak distinctly. Marty, suppose something is hurting him. Oh, God! Why doesn't he talk like everybody else?"

I couldn't believe my parents.

"He wants a crust of rye bread, Mom."

"Don't be silly, Gary . . ."

Twinkling, Marty then said, "Are you pushing rye today?"

Glenn started to cry in frustration, so I ran into the kitchen and brought out a crust of bread, which I gave him. Glenn smiled and happily gummed it.

"He was right, Marge. The kid was hungry."

"Just for *rye* bread?"

Nevertheless they stared at me in wonder. And so it was with a carrot stick, a change of diaper or a glass of milk. They weren't interchangeable, these desires or word formations, and don't ask me how I knew. The answer was that I relayed all of Glenn's requests. Whether the kid was practicing to be my stooge or I really knew that now-forgotten tongue, whenever he became agitated and emitted those strange sounds, I was called in as translator.

"*Ubbergubalee oodle.*"

"But, of course," I would smugly explain, loving my strange power. "He wants *The New York Times.*"

We really had a great act going there, and I don't know how we did it, except that I doted on him and he knew it, and that gave us something special.

When, eventually, Glenn decided to communicate with the rest of us here on earth, and he particularly wanted me, he would call "*Ahyoo!*" There was no doubt, after a while, that, like Helen Keller, who at long last associated the word *w-a-t-e-r* with the rush of cool liquid coming from a well, that Glenn had renamed me. It was certain that he wanted me, even if he called me Ahyoo.

Marty found it fascinating and considered changing my name so people would think Glenn was now speaking, but Mother was deeply troubled. She was pretty smart and so was my father; how could they have brought this dummy into the world?

It was difficult to understand why, with me yapping nonstop all day, Glenn would sit silently conjecturing and then misname his favorite person so strangely. He was getting older. He should have known better and it wasn't funny. After all, we were so close, Glenn and I, with our secret language and everything, that one would have imagined he could say Gary, an easy name. It wasn't Ethelbert or Aloysius. And then we discovered the truth. Glenn wasn't simple after all. We were.

He *was* identifying me. It was the break we'd been looking for, the Rosetta pebble. You see, I was so errant, so elusive, that my mother was constantly calling, "Gary, where *are you?*" and Glenn, hearing this all the time and then watching me rush in from somewhere in answer to the call, inferred that my name was "Are You," which we had assumed was Ahyoo. It was truly bizarre.

What a crazy little gentleman my brother was. He was already planning to be Walter Cronkite and had no time for small talk. And in Ahyoo he found a lifetime admirer.

But I didn't make life easy for Glenn. When someone in a family is struck by a serious and chronic illness, the foundation of a whole house is shaken. It's like a house of cards, one affecting the other, and, when, instead of falling in disarray, some quick architectural changes are made to bolster the structure, everything is slightly out of whack and somebody gets a bad deal. I'm afraid that Glenn got the worst of it.

Glenn has proven to be anything but backward. He's smart and slightly cuckoo, which is marvelous, and only seemingly shy. From the beginning he was selective in his relationships, evidently not needing the immense feedback I demand. He needs fewer interrelationships than I, who, at the age of two, was already a cruise director.

Of course, he's got a great wife. I envy him that. Gise is fan-

33

tastic and has the good taste to be shorter than I am, and who the hell needs a million other people when you've got that? But, Glenn seems always to have kept his own counsel. What might have been my later contribution to his personality was his intermittent rage, which would erupt for no apparent reason, work its havoc in a tantrum and then subside, not to be suspected or expected again. But it would come like a storm—out of the blue.

I had been the first child of a good marriage and for three years the wormy apple of their eye. Then came diabetes and I was made even more special. If Glenn could be only occasionally stormy, I remained the perpetual cyclone that devastated the house along with the patience of the complaining, wailing victims. Glenn was always off limits. He was in the eye of the cyclone. I would have killed for him, but the pandemonium I caused and the domination of the household by such a pretender to the throne must have touched off some of his baby ponderings, those dimpled cogitations. They may have had something to do with me and how he planned to handle it all when he had some authority and mobility.

My brother saw the effect that my needs had on Marge and Marty and he decided early to take the high road. If I was the tsetse fly, he was going to be the serum to save the family. If I would make war, then he would sue for peace. When I fought with my mother he would say—when he conquered English—

"Come on, Gary. You must know Mom is right."

So was he; but I could have throttled him. The bloody little peacemaker! Glenn loved us all and without his solace my parents would have been institutionalized.

In a sense, Glenn's thoughtful expression was my conscience but I didn't let it bother me much. At Camp Ocala in Florida—my third attempt at sleepaway camp—my reputation was so awful that my expertise came to the attention of the head counselor. He begged for my services as hitman to do in the night-watchman who had reported *him* for some after-hours infraction.

I was to fill a bucket with water, climb the roof of the bunk house, attract his attention and then drop it on the poor guy's head. I improved on the original plan. In order to fill the bucket to brimming, I rounded up the rest of the cabin who collaborated enthusiastically. Glenn felt sorry for the watchman because he was so ugly.

Glenn was always sorry for somebody. When we played cowboys and Indians he insisted on being the Indian. He was always the Confederate in our Civil Wars. He was always identifying with the underdog. I never got that message. I would have to conquer and then be kind.

# 5

W HEN GLENN SUCCEEDED me at school, a Greek chorus of horrified teachers backing off in terror chanted hoarsely, "You're not related to *Gary* Kleiman, are you?"

Glenn saved our good name. Civilized, studious and popular, he got straight A's. Day and night, we were. There aren't many children who have been expelled from kindergarten, and from then on it was downhill all the way for me.

Marge always said that I was the only boy to graduate from high school without attending it. I never studied, cut classes or upset them with my antics, was absolutely bored by the curriculum and constantly up to mischief. I was so impatient with what I believed to be the belaboring of the obvious that I couldn't or wouldn't attend. Still, I always managed at least a B and sometimes an A. There were a few teachers I respected, but few. For these rare souls I gave my all. My arrogance I did not acquire at school. It was inborn. My reluctance to attend in any sense harked back to a particularly creative instructor in elementary school.

It was law that a boy of six be schooled, so I was forced by the federal government to sit still for a period of time and learn to read, write—and ideally to evolve into a human being. Of course, I felt oppressed and my devils kept whispering terrible suggestions into my pointed ears. I had rebelled against authority at home and these people weren't even family. They didn't even feed and take care of me when I was sick or anything. But one day when I was in third grade, that particular teacher said something that riveted me to my seat. I loved language because I could articulate all the feverish thoughts that flew into my head; and I always loved words and new ideas. Well, this teacher that day said, "Children, I am going to give you a magic formula." I sat up in my seat like a Doberman about to be fed.

"I have a way," she continued, "of finding the right word in a dictionary as fast as you can say Jack Robinson."

Well, I don't think I'd ever felt such a thrill of expectancy. What a thing to discover. If that was what could happen in school, then school was for me. How neat. How truly great. I would never raise my hand to go to the boys' room unnecessarily again. I would never claim that I was having a reaction and have to lie down or leave for Fig Newtons or chocolate milk. What was this wonderful formula, this magic?

Teacher now opened the immense class dictionary and said, "Here's the trick, children. When a word begins with the letter A as in apple or arrow, what do you do? You look under the letter A and you then find out what it means. If it begins with the letter L, then you don't go to the beginning but toward the middle till you reach the L's."

I did not, could not believe that she was saying this. It wasn't to be believed. She wasn't qualified to teach a kitten to play with string. Did this educator really believe that I would meander through the whole book until on the last page I would end my search for *zebra*?

The other children were obediently copying this wisdom, this brilliant shortcut, in their notebooks and I stared at them and at her in astonishment. I then dreamed of nailing the windows shut or chalking the dumb teacher's seat or, better yet, just forging an excuse from class. I was eventually to master several important signatures. "Look under the letter A," indeed. I guess my impatience made me move ahead more quickly than the other children. I certainly felt that I was in a class by myself.

\* \* \*

Poor Glenn had to follow in my terrible wake and, for a while, I could get away with anything. Like a dutiful and elder brother, I initiated him into sports, taught him everything I knew—some of which he wisely discarded—and when on rare occasions he went into a conniption, I would hold him down and never fight back. I would just cry for help. He was totally exempt from my devilry, whatever my aggressions toward everyone else. However, I was not above making him this sorcerer's apprentice.

One summer, in order to make extra money, Glenn and I had helped paint Marty's factory's walls. I remember so well the echoing conversations we would have as we used great extension poles in these immense rooms.

"Will we ever be through . . . ever be through?" "This is the end . . . this is the end." "Good-bye forever . . . -bye forever."

And because of our exemplary work and through our father, we got a job painting the steps at an apartment complex not too far from home. I got my act together, and Glenn, a friend named Dave Rhonda and I drove over and did the best we could, which was terrible. The man who hired us, however, was more interested in thrift than quality and then asked us to paint the outside concrete balconies of the apartments. They had wrought-iron posts—tough as hell to paint.

We were having a really hot spell, and the color the landlord had chosen was bile—I mean a terrible green. Now there is really no quick way of painting that kind of balustrade, but we tried several. It was like a Chaplin or Laurel and Hardy clip. There were so many balconies and so many posts, I lost all patience. The more we patched, the worse it became. There was no way of cleaning up the mess. After a while the building looked as if it had been sick. I mean, really offensive. I decided that three was a crowd and from that day on—with the ghost of Huck Finn prompting me—I drove Glenn and Dave to work every day, went about my business and then returned to collect them and a percentage of the loot. After all, I had gotten them the job. These experiences certainly helped Glenn grow up.

I, however, still seemed not to be growing at all. At school the boys towered over me and the girls thought me cute instead of magnificent. I wasn't in the least cute. I delivered newspapers—I had a paper route for a while—but my employer made the mistake of paying me in advance. I was in serious danger of becoming a real hood.

I then got a job as a busboy at The Carriage House, a restaurant that paid me a dollar and a quarter an hour and ten percent of any tips, plus anything I could cadge from the customers for just being adorable. This was one of the low points in a life whose terrain is not known for its mountain peaks. I had to wear a smock that was the uniform of the place, and their smallest available size was so large that I was swamped in it. No amount of pinning, rolling or gluing kept me from looking like one of Disney's Seven. It was mortifying as well as clumsy. I was always tripping, spilling or breaking something as all that loose material swept everything before it. I loved making people laugh, but on *my* terms and with my own material. I shudder still at my embarrassment and the hilarity my appearance inspired.

Glenn had already caught up with me, was already my size, and had to his delight at last reached puberty. Marge, who seemed to have sensed the exact moment, chose to have another sex talk with both of us. It is incredible that she found this one subject absolutely impossible to discuss with any degree of intelligence, clarity or sanity. I guess she thought we were about to impregnate all the daughters of her friends.

"Now listen, Glenn—sit still, Gary, and hear this—I know boys will be boys and I'm not old-fashioned. I know a man should be experienced, and you're going to have to get experience, but—well—don't get experience, don't do it, with nice girls."

Since I thought all girls were nice, I was confused. I was already halfway out of the room.

"Who should we do it with, Mom—kangaroos?"

Neither of us was into the sex scene yet. Glenn was busy garnering scholastic honors being editor of the school paper and cleansing the name of Kleiman; and I, far from drooling over girls, was dribbling feverishly on our basketball courts. But we did know, Glenn and I, this much: That we should never do it with nice girls and never under any circumstances in our mother's bed. With this sex education digested, we pursued our individual interests.

I loved the teamwork of basketball, the friendship, the joint effort. And I loved being good at something. I looked like the team's mascot, however, and good as I might have been, my fleetness couldn't compensate for you know what. I was five feet tall and less than one hundred pounds; during the trials Warren Walk, all-state center—at six feet six inches—turned to me and said, "Hey, my shit is bigger than you are."

That sort of remark made "good things come in small packages" kind of forgettable.

When I tried out for the junior varsity team, I was rejected. Reluctantly, I believe. I was the very last guy to be cut. I cried and switched to tennis that evening. Hearing my tragic news, Marty took me immediately to Henderson Park to play a couple of sets.

"How about taking some lessons?" he asked offhandedly.

A family friend had already spoken to my tennis coach, who recommended me to E. John Harbett, the tennis pro at Henderson. He had suggested that I was a natural, a sleeper. Mr. Harbett now looked me over and, hallelujah, took me on.

Marge would have been delighted to know that tennis, not her friends' daughters, became my overriding passion. Running, dashing, jumping, leaping with a purpose and being healthy with other healthy people allowed me more than ever to deny my diabetes. And I wasn't too short for tennis.

As a matter of fact, things were happening and I was creeping up. There seems little doubt that diabetes had stunted my growth for years, perhaps even limiting its potential. At any rate, I was riding higher now. I was wild about tennis and lived for it. It was true I was a natural. It is also true that a talent for something is not enough, but only the beginning.

Slim Harbett made a real fat mark on my life. He not only

taught me the game, but he helped me grow up. His tennis formula was fourfold:

1. Keep arms straight but not stiff.
2. Turn sideways to the net.
3. Keep the racket above the wrist.
4. Follow through forty-five degrees above where you want the ball to land.

Great. But my impatience made me a compulsive singles player. I'd go too quickly for the kill. I burned to win at all costs, and the promise of a set would go up in smoke. I was a nervous wreck who was playing against myself. All of this Slim set about to change, but I had a lot of temperament to overcome.

When I was going strong, in eleventh grade and bouncing around the court like a winner, I called Slim one day to check our next appointment. I got, as they say, the shock of my life.

"Laddie," he said very slowly, which was his way with everything. "I think we'd better forget the next appointment. In fact, I think we'd better forget all the next appointments."

"I don't understand, Slim. What's happened? What do you mean?"

"I've been thinking about it, and it's not going well, laddie."

"You mean I'm no good? You mean I'll never make it?"

"I mean you can't control yourself, so how can you control your racket or anything?"

"Slim I—"

"You blame the sun in your eyes, the wind from the north; you blame everything but yourself. You're a spoiled kid, a paranoid."

I hung up and drove out to see him as fast as I could. I wanted to present my case and then plead it. I listened instead.

"There is no situation and no combination of circumstances that you can't conquer. I believe this and I want you to believe it. If you face yourself and you make up your mind to take the responsibility, if you *stop blaming everyone else*—"

By the time Slim Harbett's candor and his "strength philosophy" had driven home some truths to me, he had me playing doubles at Miami Beach High and ranking, along with my partner, Brooks Kurtz, twelfth in the state.

He saw to it that I was on my way. Doubles really was my game. The interplay, the feedback. With a partner I became better than good. And yet it was me. I could dropshot and lob and slice with the best of them. My backhand was just fair, my forehand good and my serve spectacular. I could change pace, vary the spins. Jesus, I love tennis. I used to play a lot with Janet Haas, who never lost a match in her entire high school tennis career, 69–0. She went on to the University of Miami, the Virginia Slims-sponsored tournament and then to Wimbledon. I met Chrissie Evert through her, and we all played Henderson and North Shore parks. Chrissie, who doesn't need my endorsement, could place a ball, even early on, within a fraction of an inch of its mark. Christ! I saw her at Forest Hills years later and she melted at the sight of an old tennis bum from back home.

"God! Those were the good old days," she said wistfully, which made me wonder.

Janet Haas was, to me, a great all-around athlete. We met first at the Roney Plaza pool when we were about five or six and she was doing a backflip off the highest board. She's still fearless. We played a lot of great and crazy tennis together at Flamingo, North Shore and Henderson parks, and we toured the state in tournaments. Her friendship, never once faltering, her breezy, bluff, no-crap affection is duly noted. To me, she's Diana. And I mean the original one.

But it was that grizzled, weather-beaten tall Scot, Slim Harbett, with his old tar's tanned face shaded with an ancient white tennis hat, who really whipped me into shape. He once had used the expression "Smother Mother" about another pupil's devouring parent, and I all too quickly had adapted it for my own private use. Smother Mother! That was Marge to me. I obviously was fighting my battle with her—often shadowboxing—twenty-four hours a day. And it had started at the outset.

Even before the diabetes, we had chosen our corners. I actually remember being in my crib and, of course, wanting out. I was born with the wanderlust. Half is memory, half family legend. All of it true. I wanted to be picked up, I guess, or allowed to go places, and didn't quite have the necessary credentials to make the decision. My mother thought it time for me to sleep. "Uh-uh!"

I yelled and coughed and cried and Marge was having none of it. She was doing the Brahms bit, and I was in no mood for lullabies. I repeated my scene ever louder, but Marge stuck to her guns. It was Kleiman versus Kleiman and I got out the real ammunition. I banged my lip against the side of the crib so hard that blood gushed all over the quilt. Needless to report, I was removed from the crib. The decision was mine.

I would have my way. I was committed to eternal battle with this glamorous woman who would thwart my efforts. There was a string of preliminaries that had to do with late hours, use of public buses, intransigence at school and utter anarchism at home. My father was a sometime ally when he recognized my greater need for some independence, and Marge lengthened the leash slowly but perceptibly as I grew older.

I didn't always remember that over the healthy, uneventful years, I still had been hospitalized a few times, that my silent, hidden condition did make me vulnerable and my personality problems did not promise prudence.

I was still playing it both ways in school, demanding special treatment and wanting to be treated as if I were healthy. I could get away with murder, the teachers were so intimidated. They seemed to be delighted by me, but only until I was in their classes. Yet, they did find it difficult to be too harsh for fear something would happen to me. I thought I had it made.

The best-laid plans of little boys, etcetera, etcetera. One day, while running around the classroom—in about fourth grade—I tripped and fell. Always cued in to make the most of a situation, I decided to fake a leg injury so I could be excused. Now my diabetes was, of course, necessarily known about by the faculty at school, but there was no need to broadcast it. This well-meaning, unthinking teacher took me to the nurse. When he returned to the class, he seems to have gone bonkers. He announced that Gary was a very sick boy and went on to describe diabetes as a combination of hemophilia and leprosy. Absolutely ignorant of the disease, he frightened the kids into feeling that a pat on my back could be fatal. When I heard what he had done, *I* went crazy. He had made me a freak to my classmates, and I couldn't face them I was so mortified.

It was such an unbelievable thing to do. The worst. At the clinic, the first thing we avoid is making a child feel unattractive or dangerous to be with. This burden is greater than the sickness. It's unbearable. The teacher's betrayal bore the expected fruit. In the playground a short time later, one of the kids I'd always played and roughhoused with crouched in terror.

"Keep away from him," he yelled to everybody. "He has diabetes and you can catch it."

All the kids backed off slowly, retreating to the four corners of the yard until I was standing alone in the middle of it. I stood there raging, holding back the tears and having to pee desperately. I must have resembled a dried up version of Brussels's famous little boy. I stood my ground until recess was over and then ran all the way home, unable in any way to contain myself. I flung myself at my mother, who tried to calm me. Later, she and Marty suggested that the following day I patiently explain the facts of my life to the crazy little bastard. That I enlighten him. And it all worked out exactly as they said it would. The kid listened, I mean really interested, and then apologized.

Some kids had to be handled differently, however. At the water fountain one morning, some mean-looking nerd looked up, saw I was next on line and, hogging the water, still pressing the faucet and giving himself what looked like an ear syringe, snarled, "Look who's here. How about coming up with a coma for us today?"

I went berserk. He and several others who got in the way were on the floor. No one was safe around me. I became a spitting machine gun. I was almost expelled.

These were my healthy, normal years and I wore a tag around my neck like a dog. Only mine read:

MY NAME IS GARY KLEIMAN
I AM A DIABETIC
IF WEAK OR DIZZY, PLEASE
GIVE ME SUGAR, CANDY, JUICE
OR SODA. (*Over*)

*Over!* It was mortifying. On the flip side of this record of a normal child was my address and telephone number, along with the name of my doctor. Is it any wonder that the diabetic wants to deny the illness—even the reactions themselves? Some of us have *refused* to react in order to avoid a scene. This is, of course, insanity, because it only becomes worse. But we try to will it away. This public and unattractive display of helplessness, the fear that at any time it may occur is a nightmare.

We are walking groceries as well as drug stores. We don't dare go anywhere without candy bars, sugar cubes, or sodas. At the first signs of queasiness one can usually avoid the oncoming debilitation but not always. We must always be prepared.

If we are caught without these compensating sweets and our sugar level drops too severely, we can reel, tremble, fall and even black out. It's like being in a zoo if you are private in grief and illness. But one can't be private with diabetes. You lose consciousness on a pavement with a circle of curious but unfeeling eyes watching your descent like a half-attentive, popcorn munching movie audience. I may love attention but not this kind.

Now Marge knew all of this and with her lively imagination knew even more. How could she protect me? To hear her tell it, she was always holding her breath as she let me go my way as she knew she must. Am I really only remembering the times she didn't? Is she only remembering the times she did? And am I still so programmed that I belabor the past, hoping to be free of all restrictions, especially those so recently added?

*45*

All I know is that my mother's searchlight eyes—most feeling and most attentive—were always seeking out the dusty corners of my restive spirit. And she's a great housekeeper. I believe it was the Chinese who observed "Every child should be beaten once a day. If you don't know the reason why, he does."

# 6

I STARTED turning into a human being when I was about six-teen, although my parents wouldn't have agreed. It wasn't a complete transformation but it was a beginning. I was playing tennis and since I had always loved drawing I was studying art in school. Again I was a natural and was encouraged and somewhat domesticated by my teacher, Lloyd Slone, whose enthusiasm fired me. Although he was always encouraging, he could be tough with me.

Mr. Slone frankly told me that I simply wasn't realizing my potential and I was goofing around. I always wanted to do things my own way. First, I avoided figure drawings of which I was not too sure and then, when conquered, clouds and oceans. I was learning that people outside my family evidently were not going to take my crap. It was hard to believe. But I still loved drawing and I sought approval. I also remembered Slim. By the time I was through, I had become art editor of the school yearbook and won Dade County's Silver Knight senior award in art, which was a kind of Oscar and something that not only made me proud but further encouraged me to think seriously about a career in art.

Though I was still unpredictable, I was no longer a wild cell totally unconscious of my surroundings and often destructive of them. Perhaps a bit late, I was growing up. I was still immature, but I liked women and was thinking about them a lot and in a more specific way. I knew, however, that I was on safer ground with my fellow jocks. Both my thoroughly modern parents were apparently embarrassed to discuss the particulars of sex with me, and, in this regard only, we might have been a Bible-fearing seventeenth-century Plymouth family. The tone had been set and I was as Puritan as they, but my instincts originated even earlier and so I took the plunge.

My friend Steve Carlin and I were driving up to Gainesville to see some friends at the University of Florida and we decided to go to Daytona and seek adventure. I was sixteen and looked eleven. Cocky as I was, I had my doubts as well as desires. We cruised around and at last picked up two girls who turned out to be thirteen. Like experienced and kindly fishermen, we threw them back. I breathed a sigh of relief. Our next two got in the car and were so spaced out on drugs that we chickened out and dumped them at the next corner. I was having the best of two possible worlds; I was being a man about town and not having to put it on the line. These disastrous encounters were both burnishing my image and saving my face.

"Hi! Do you want a ride?" Steve shouted with growing authority to two others.

I was myself leering at one of them—a beautiful older woman, probably past her teens. I knew she would put me in my place if she noticed me at all. I could barely be seen above the window.

"Pull over," this long-haired, long-legged foxy lady commanded. I thought she was going to swat me. This was great—playing with fire and wearing asbestos gloves. We did as she directed.

"How about a lift, boys?" she asked. "We're on our way to Miami and been hitching our way from Virginia. Well? How about it?"

"OK," Steve said, "but we're not leaving till morning."

The girls looked at each other and then at us.

"That's OK. Just fine."

My heart pounded as they climbed into the car with their

bags. I was committed now; and gritting my teeth, I almost bit my heart. After a hamburger, we drove back to our motel, both of us guys breathing heavily.

"I want the one with the long hair," I whispered, not sure that anything was really going to happen but demanding the winner anyway.

"You gotta be kidding," Steve muttered. "The other one has a mustache."

I had noticed.

"That's more than we have," I answered.

"Well, let's just see where they go," tall, handsome Steve said with what was designed to sound like absolute fairness.

Women are so marvelous. While the girls fussed around in the bathroom, Steve and I got into bed and nervously awaited them. I didn't have a chance, but I prayed and Mary came to me. Thank God—she must have had a mother thing or something because she walked into the room, smiled and came straight to me. They must have been doing some talking, too. Steve was disappointed. I was not.

I might have been short, but I rose to the occasion. Through sheer desire, instinct and brass, I prevailed. It was my world premiere. Even though I wasn't back at home in Marge's bed, I still felt guilty. I wasn't supposed to be in Daytona. I had just had sex with a girl I had "met" and Mary was certainly *nice*. Though I couldn't have been more elated, it was a new, bizarre and kind of tacky scene, sharing this ugly room. I guess I was a little squeamish.

We, all of us, for whatever reason, awoke with group paranoia at the scream of an ambulance siren during the night. We ran naked to the window, hearts thumping and convinced that the FBI, the vice squad and our parents were coming to get us.

When morning did come, I got up before the rest, of course, and picked my own pocket, filching my syringe and insulin. I crept into the bathroom, gave myself my first shot of the day, returned the objects and then rejoined sleeping Mary so I could "awaken" as carefree as the others.

With the mystery of women solved, I'd found another outlet for my energy. But I was a romantic who wanted much more than a night in a motel. In some misty future I vaguely imagined a faceless, marvelous girl with whom I would make a happy, hilarious marriage and have bouncing, healthy tennis-playing sons. There was a lot of love stored up inside me, and at home I had the perfect example of how to lavish it. The dream might have been vague, undetailed, but I dreamed of a marriage just like Marge and Marty's. I was still able to dream at seventeen.

I don't kid myself any longer. And I won't kid anyone else. Like, I mean, right now, though I think I'll be going home—certainly not to my own apartment at first, but to my family's house—I'm going to be as fragile as glass for a while. For the rest of my life I'll be a slave to doctors and prescribed self-indulgence. Could I ask a woman to share this? And what kind of a woman would want to? She'd have to be out of her ever-loving—in which case why would I want her? It's like Groucho's distress and disenchantment with the country club that decided to accept the likes of him.

A husband is not supposed to be fragile, medicating, testing all day, at hospitals three times a week, all mobility gone, always on the alert for the worst. A woman would have to be out of her head.

No matter how I dissemble, laugh and fight it, the truth of the matter is that I am always dependent on someone else, fetched and delivered like a fucking parcel. With no sovereignty. I haven't in the recent past even been able to call the finish to a social evening or casual relationship. Unlike other guys, I couldn't, if I felt it desirable or even necessary to split, take it on the lam, leave in a huff. I can't love 'em and leave 'em and I can't love 'em forever either.

Way back when I was a senior in high school, I did meet a special girl named Robin. She was a friend of someone I was dating. I was too dumb or smart to have recognized a person I could be serious about, and so I kept my distance and watched her from afar. Since my Daytona triumph, I had been scoring between basketball and tennis games, but I didn't have the foggiest of how to be a "boyfriend," a committed half of a unit. I was emotionally about three years old.

She was unattached then, but I did nothing about it. We did, eventually, become friends, and I enjoyed her company. I also enjoyed looking at her hazel eyes, her long fair hair, her cute bangs and that smile. But before I graduated to any real relationship, I miraculously got through high school.

When Marty took me up to his alma mater, Syracuse, in my senior year to see if I was interested in enrolling, I felt not only that I was going to start a new chapter in my life—a nice, new fresh slate, a great new adventure—but I also had a warming notion that there was still another dimension to my life and there would someday—maybe soon—be someone I would be thinking about a lot, someone who might really care for me. There were hints and glints of something golden we might share in the misty future.

# 7

I T WAS fascinating seeing my father's reaction to the scenes of his youth. He had loved college, had gone ape over Syracuse and had filled me with rollicking tales of collegiate life. He wanted me to enjoy the "best years of one's life" as he had. Wouldn't you know he'd been Joe College, an old rah-rah guy? He had been a real campus nut, even painting his shoes orange in his freshman zeal. A real Boy From Syracuse.

As fine looking and chipper as Marty was in 1971, he wasn't eighteen since I was; and there on the wintry campus with lots of pink-faced kids whirling around through the snow, I think he saw his own ghost. The return only lengthened the distance of the past. His ready grin seemed, as everything else that February, a bit frozen. It was fascinating. It was sad. But it was my turn now he said; and that replenished him. He could relive it through me.

Now that I was going to enter college what did I want to study beside hellraising for which I had already won an honorary degree? If I'd thought of a profession at all, if ever I were asked what I wanted to be as a grown-up, I always answered, "a veterinarian." I saw myself as aging, kindly, short and lovable Doc Kleiman with a black bag, a convertible and a menagerie of smiling dumb creatures encircling me in adoration and gratitude for my unpaid services. My love of animals and our doctor-patient relationship made Drs. Doolittle and Herriot look like vivisectionists.

It was not to be. It seemed that veterinary medicine, as all others, required math and science both of whose disciplines did not attract me.

My other love was architecture and I believe that I have brought a feeling for it to my work; but its upper reaches were similarly impossible to reach without a successful negotiation of its foundations. My impatience wanted nothing less than instant gratification. With four years ahead of me and a simple bachelor of arts demanding subjects I felt beyond me, my interview seemed doomed.

The dean was a kind man with small eyes and gigantic hands; and when Marty, aware of both my gifts and my shortcomings, suggested that I enroll in the art school, we were all delighted. The dean informed me that I would have to get together a portfolio by April and I promised I would. When I got home I knocked out forty pieces—paintings, drawings, watercolors—all in one week.

I had designed the cover of the Miami Beach High School yearbook, so I photographed it and added it to the collection. I was really with it, raring to go. It was all coming together. April, hell. I sent on the portfolio immediately, and practically by return mail the university accepted me.

Just to prove that I could do it, I got straight A's in that last semester in high school and made the honor roll twice. Marge and Marty were struck dumb. It was the only year in which they were not called to school because of my behavioral problems. I had also dropped a lot of dudes who hung around the shopping mart at Miami Beach's Lincoln Road Mall. We did nothing but watch the girls go by, listen to records and look like hoods.

Marge was sure that we were up to something terrible. It was worse. We were up to nothing, completely. We swarmed in and out of the five-and-ten and the supermarket and clothing stores like sheep, huddled together and nonthinking. I don't remember one intelligent thought being shared. I guess it was enough that we were *mucho* macho.

I soon got bored, bought a guitar and made music with another group. Thank God, I'm my own pot and never needed anything to stir me up. Anyway, sports were still most exciting to me, so I found myself with a younger, less worldly group. I never made any dramatic change. I greeted everybody with a warm "hi," but I remember calling myself Switzerland in those days. I was the neutral zone, allied to no particular gang, not bottled with any label. I had always wanted—I *have* always wanted—to be unique and treated as an individual with special needs and demands. Being part of any rat pack was not my style.

Marty had recalled his old fraternity house with great feeling. I was sure that I wouldn't want to join one. It was still Gary Kleiman against the world. And that world was now going to expand.

The whole family took me to the airport when I left for Syracuse and Glenn—I couldn't believe it—gave me a lecture.

"I know college is going to change you, Gary. Please—don't let it."

He was sure that I was going to come home a dope addict. I was sure we were going to miss each other.

My father never lectures. He wanted me to make a "fresh start," which now sounds as if I was leaving the penitentiary for more promising days, and in a way I was. My mother's vigil was over. There was nothing she could have said or not said that wouldn't have put me on edge. Those were particularly tense days in our relationship. She got the brunt of everything. If she had said what Marty then said, "Have fun!" I would have accepted it as a crack, a prophesy of pleasure-seeking laziness; and I would have read into it a sarcasm that would have provoked a vicious reply. When Marty said it, I knew he was hoping I would relish my youth and do him the favor of replacing him as campus cutup.

It is interesting how, as we grow older, we discover that what people say is not as important as how we listen. We heed what we will and, even with my father's joyous send-off, I knew that he wanted me—with that fresh start—to get with it.

When I looked out of the window of the plane on that gray day, I saw my mother just as she put on her sunglasses and turned to wave. "She's crying," I said to myself in irritation. "How typical. *Mothers!* It's great to be getting away from all this crap." I knew she was hiding tears. But if she had waved and I'd seen them, I would have been equally annoyed, and if she hadn't cried, I would have been furious that she was always in such control.

Freedom. To be eighteen and off to college, and since my life was one long vacation without pay, I was also going to stop off first with a cousin and see the matches at Forest Hills. It was too much. I was, as I flew north, on top of the world.

I was off to college and Chris Evert was off to the big time. At sixteen she was playing her first tournament in Forest Hills—against Billie Jean King. I had to be there, remembering that incredible, two-fisted backhand and that blond, bobbing ponytail. For a tennis player she was really cute. She was also a quiet, strictly reared, very correct student at St. Thomas Aquinas. She and Janet Haas used to play a lot along with Laurie Fleming, all of them great friends down in Miami. Now she was determined to conquer Long Island for a starter.

I was caught up in the excitement as I saw Pancho Gonzales, in the middle of a traffic jam, zigzagging through the street waving twelve rackets, banging on the hoods of cars, yelling for everybody to "Move!" He was acting exactly like Pancho Gonzales and I loved it.

He was there putting on a serving demonstration with Margaret Smith Court. The crowds were immense, but I got into the clubhouse thanks to Gardnar Mulloy, an old buddy from Henderson Park. It was then that I found Chris. I just stood there with folded arms as she looked up from a plate of food and caught sight of me.

"What are *you* doing here?" she asked.

It was a real double take.

"Well, I heard about a kid from Fort Lauderdale—a lot of noise about her—so I decided to see for myself."

And I saw plenty after I took my seat. She was just wonderful. I heard someone yell, "It's a long way from Henderson Park," and it was another kid from Miami. I got a terrific, warm feeling, and then I saw a few more faces from down home, all of them there to cheer the girl on. It was really nice and I loved being a part of it.

It was a golden kind of day, and knowing when it was over that I, too, was starting a new chapter of my life, I shared in the excitement more than vicariously. I had never seen grass courts before and I guess I wondered, yes, wondered, in the general euphoria, if I'd ever play on them myself. Why not?

Yep! I was flying and eventually made a three-point landing in Syracuse, where my roommate, Artie, picked me up in his van. He proudly showed me everything and in no time flat I'd seen the Mount, Flint and Day Hall and been briefed about a chick named Betty with hair down to her ankles. It was really great—all of it. And promising.

When I saw our room and the bed which I hadn't been given an opportunity to choose, I knew some redecoration was in order. Artie and I redid the whole shebang with bunk beds over our desks and a burlap divider. When we got through it was a palace compared to the other dorms. I guess we were the spoiled rich kids from Florida, with our own phone and everything. I loved it. Best of all, no one was watching over me. The microscope was fifteen hundred miles away.

Of course, I brought my own problems to Freedom Hall. I was safe with Artie. I had chosen him for a roommate because he knew my story and was a responsible guy who wasn't going to use my needles and freak out on heroin, presenting me with serum hepatitis as well as everything else. In case I had trouble, he also could handle the situation.

But I was no longer a big frog, Glenn's older brother racing around in his Camaro reluctantly sold before I went north. A big shot in my senior year. I was starting all over again in a new place: still short, still wanting it all my way, denying my illness, but at first opportunity buying a car and getting a medical sticker for it. I always managed the special privileges.

I loved Syracuse, despite the weather, which rivals Buffalo

and the Yukon. The oldness, the Gothic architecture, the crisp clear air and the music and laughter coming from all the dorms. I loved the excitement and the fact that my friend Sergio Mendes from Miami was urging me to join the tennis team. But I was unsure of myself. I really do not exaggerate. I still looked about eleven. It was obscene. The guys and especially the girls would gaze at me with mouths agape. I wasn't even shaving at eighteen.

"You mean you're *attending* this college?"

"May I ask how *old* you are, buster?"

"Hey, are you some kind of quiz kid or something?"

Down home, I had become a familiar sight. In a small town, a two-headed creature eventually passes unnoticed. But here, I had to start all over again. Keeping my temper, earning some respect, proving myself. In Miami Beach my proudest possession and my only escape was my automobile. My wonderful green Camaro with the dark green top. How I loved that car and the license it afforded me.

Sometimes when Marge and Marty thought I was up to something terrible, I was just driving by myself along the water, part of the elements, almost in an ecstasy. I kept one hand over my face so that drivers who passed me (when I allowed it) couldn't bore me with their surprised, "Does your mother know you've traded your kiddy car for this great big car?" or, "When does Florida give a kid a license—when he's six?"

But when I was alone, unbothered, aware that the path of the sun or moon on the water was sticking with me like a buddy while the palm trees slipped and swayed past me, when I felt the power beneath my foot and had control of time and space, I was wonderfully happy—suspended between places and obligations and indignities.

I started art classes but, as usual, play came first. Tennis took first priority and both Sergio and I made varsity, which thrilled me. That kind of encouragement was essential to me. But no one knew how I was going to reconcile my drawing classes with sports. I didn't.

As for art, if it wasn't exactly the big time I was in, I had to confess that for the first time I was not the best in the class. Some of these guys were really serious and also terribly intellectual about their approach to a piece of drawing paper; it was easy for me to mock them. But, Jesus, they were good. I tried addressing myself to their self-consciousness, their ever-so-cosmic approach to everything from a conte crayon to a life-class model's ass. I laughed at all their *artsy-shmartsy* jazz and yawned at their critiques, always severe and terribly existential, and I wouldn't meet their challenge. I cranked out what the professors demanded and no more. If I didn't really try, I couldn't be found wanting.

This is what I was doing with girls. It's what I was doing with everything. I was glib. I was fast. And so I settled for adequacy. I had thought vaguely, if I thought at all, that I might go into advertising, industrial art, maybe even landscape architecture— drawing trees, designing golf courses—ignoring the figure that I was having a more difficult time with now.

There was a girl, Stacy, who looked at my work one day and really laced into me. She was always direct. When she first saw me she really cracked up.

"You're Puck," she screamed. "You're not for real."

This was a variation at least. Now she looked over one of my latest drawings.

"This stinks," she said.

"Thank you," I replied.

"But you can do so much better than that, Puck. If you'd just *try*! If you couldn't, I wouldn't say anything. This is crap."

She was tough, she was great, but I quickly changed into my tennis things and dashed off.

One of my professors—in general drawing—had complimented me on my work. I knew my grade was between an A and a B, and when the marks were posted and I'd gotten a B, I confronted him with this outrage.

"I don't understand, Professor Dresher. You told me back a bit that I was in between the two grades. Why did you give me a B?"

"Because when you first started in my class you were the best."

"And so . . ."

"And so you started sliding—backward."

"Why didn't you say something."

"I didn't think I had to."

"But you're the teacher. You're supposed to teach."

"You'll do fine, Kleiman, if you just draw what you see and stop trying to please me."

"Fine. Now will you give me an A? Now? Why can't you do that?" I grinned winningly.

"Because I want you to earn it. I want you to try!"

I decided that I would really try. If I really had to work to get this A, then work it would be.

"OK, Professor, I promise I'll get that A the next time around."

In the interim there were endless hours of fun! Sports and clowning always gave me a sense of superiority. People accepted me as a jock or a clown. I seemed able to relate primarily on those levels without loss of face, and I didn't discuss diabetes with anyone except the faculty. But people knew.

There was one crazy, wonderful guy named Tom Fairchild who always wore a Stetson. He was as nutty as I and open as all Texas. He came into my dorm one night and point-blank asked it. And in front of some other guys.

"What actually *is* diabetes, Gar? Do you mind if I ask?"

"No. I want you to. Great."

"Then tell us all about it. What is it exactly and how do you handle it?"

They all sat around in a circle like medical students as I explained the symptoms, the medications and the diet.

"Then why do you drink all this Coke you've got all around the place?" Tom asked.

Good question. I parried by telling them about reactions and the need for sweets when my sugar level is dangerously low, but they were not fools.

"But won't it go too high with such excess?"

"Yes, it will," I answered, making a promise to myself that I would cut back.

I remember having uncommon headaches during this period and attributing them to some English exams. Coke seemed to make me feel better. No one ever bothered to note that I was still drinking them after that and that was fine, because I was sure I had everything under control. I surely didn't want any Marges peeking into my refrigerator—another privilege I was allowed because of my condition.

Anyway, this confidence helped me become closer to the guys. A few of them became real buddies. I clinched it one night when, while some were drunk and others spaced out, I suddenly said, "Let's do something crazy. I mean, real crazy."

"OK, Gary, like what?"

"Oh, I don't know."

I was thinking fast. I had everybody's attention and I wasn't going to lose it.

"What about condemning the Hall of Languages?"

The Hall of Languages was the oldest and most venerated building at Syracuse. HL we called it. They looked at me as if I were totally bonkers, but they were fascinated. It was marvelous being in charge—even if it was a black mass. My enthusiasm was infectious. Everybody's eyes lighted up as I improvised.

Under my expert tutelage, we became the Hood Patrol. We dressed in lumberjack hats and black gloves, putting black shoe polish all over our faces. Led by Tom and me, we boarded up the whole building using lumber that was being stored for library reconstruction. We stenciled the word CONDEMNED all over the walls, windows and doors with orange paint I contributed. Through a series of signals, we eluded the night watchman and completely got away with it.

After successfully blocking the forces of education, we retired to my room for a libation and self-applause. It was then that Tom told me about isopropyl alcohol, which I use every day for my shots but whose other advantages were unknown to me.

"You mean you didn't know," Tom asked, "that you can light the stuff and the flames won't burn you?"

We sat enchanted as he demonstrated. He applied the isopropyl on his hand and painlessly set it on fire!

"Will this work on wood? On people's doors?" I asked.

"I told you. Only the alcohol will burn. Nothing will even char."

"It isn't really dangerous, just scary, huh?"

"Right."

I then covered my RA's door with the stuff, knocked, set the door aflame and scooted. The kid was almost frightened out of his senses; he didn't think it was at all funny. I was beside myself.

At Christmas, I went home like a conquering hero—the college man, ready to set the world on fire.

Marty was doing really well at this point. I mean, his business was thriving and nothing was too good for all of us. I just picked up and surprised everyone by coming home for the Dolphins-Baltimore Colts game. I wasn't supposed to return until intersession, which was after final exams some weeks later, but the playboy took both trips. The second one was crucial. I got a cold, a bad one. It turned into the flu and my fever soared.

A girl I had been seeing in high school for a little while had not readily accepted the end of our unimportant romance. I was back in town and hadn't called her. It was Robin, that special girl at high school I telephoned and she sounded weird, preoccupied, I was certain, with someone else. I was piqued. But this other gal was upset because I hadn't telephoned and had disappeared. Some friends buzzed to tell me and then—there I was in bed sick—the girl's mother telephoned demanding to know if she was with me. This was ridiculous and I said so. The woman was desperate and I got out of bed and joined two other friends to find her—at Fun Fair, Coconut Grove—all over the place. It was madness my being out and I was getting dizzier and wearier all night.

The next morning I was so bad that I had to be hospitalized. It was my second bout with DKA—diabetic ketoacidosis—an evil liver secretion of acids into the bloodstream and disastrous dehydration. The first one was at day camp when I was thirteen and entirely due to neglect, self-indulgence and denial. I wanted to prove I could do anything and not get sick. Yeah! Sure. This time it was out of my control.

The lost young lady called the hospital guiltily. She'd been found and now felt responsible for my illness. Chances are that I would have landed there anyway—perhaps not so soon but surely.

The doctors told us not to worry but they'd found a trace of albumin—a little protein in my urine. This occurs when there is kidney deterioration but many people have a trace without dire results. Diabetics, however, must beware. This was January of 1972. It was about to hit the fan.

# 8

FULLY RECOVERED from the flu, I wanted to buy a new car to drive back to Syracuse, and my choice was a Datsun. The new one was just out, but Marty preferred my having a heavier car, Ford's Gran Torino sport, and this time he prevailed.

Sergio Mendes and I drove it back to Syracuse in twenty-six hours. While I was driving, I had a couple of hours of fatigue which seemed to blur my vision slightly. I even thought it was the fog once we reached Pennsylvania. Exhausted when we arrived at college, I fell into bed.

Before I'd left the hospital, I'd been given the name of an endocrinologist in Syracuse and advised to check in to make sure all was well. Since it was wise to have a doctor up there anyway, I made an appointment on February ninth. I felt fine but I didn't want a repeat performance of the flu or DKA.

My tennis game, as a result of them, seemed shaky. It was, I suspected, the aftermath of fever. But when we started to have our intramural basketball games I decided I had to get a new prescription for my glasses. One night, sitting with Artie—studying and listening to some Simon and Garfunkel, I looked up and saw waves and ripples in the air. It was almost as if the air had turned somewhat substantial, like chiffon.

"Jesus, the heater must be going full blast," I said. But it wasn't even turned on. Then I looked at the album cover and *it* was blurred.

"Why in God's name do it out of focus? Is this supposed to be arty?" And then I blinked and Artie looked at me questioningly. Everything became sharp again and I said, "I've got to get new glasses. Poring over these damned books and drawings is straining my eyes."

Artie was rarely sleeping in the room. His girl friend had switched from Penn State and he now had a lovelier roommate. And so, when Glenn came up to visit his big brother and to see college life, he stayed with me for a marvelous weekend.

Glenn had never before seen snow and got lost in the drifts. I mean, really disappeared a couple of times.

I showed him everything and we went to the Syracuse-U of Mass basketball game.

"Jesus, it's foggy in here, Glenn."

"What are you talking about?"

"All that smoke. Jesus."

"What smoke?"

I was playing basketball one afternoon and I passed the ball to a teammate, Jeff Southwick, up at the post. I headed to the corner where I was to catch his pass and then make my shot for the basket. I got to the corner, pumped, jumped and pawed the air. I ran back up the court and Jeff, breathless, asked what had happened. I didn't know. The solo, "What's wrong with you, Kleiman?" became a chorus on both the basketball and the tennis courts as I kept inexplicably missing targets. I rationalized my tennis off game, because it was the first indoor court I had ever played on. The ceiling kept getting in the way somehow, looming ever nearer. The blue sky was the usual roof over my lobs. I refused to face the walls that were closing in on me either. My appointment was for the ninth and until then, Glenn and I had a ball.

A whole crowd of us stole trays from the school cafeteria and used them to sleigh down the icy slope at Thorndon Park. We had a real Olympic traying session that was a hoot—and silver beautiful with all the snow and frost. It was dangerous, too, and

Tom Fairchild, whose bravery apparently ran the whole thermo-metric gamut, who never burned his hand with the isopropyl flame, now didn't freeze or break his ass on these runs, which he did, so help me, standing up. Some booze helped us to be sure, but at least the guys weren't naked this particular day. It was wild. Steering, or the attempt at steering, made you go through your gloves as if they were paper. And the speed! That slope was practically perpendicular. That ice was glass. We made our own Olympic teams and Glenn and I represented Florida with some distinction.

My brother valiantly kept climbing back up the great hill for more, but each trip was taking him longer, and I kept watching, concerned. Suddenly he staggered and fell into the snow, which sat apart every few feet or so like powder puffs on a mirror. I saw his hand reach for his asthma spray, and when I reached him, he was wheezing badly. We raced him back to the dorm, where he took further medication and rested while I made the mistake of putting my frostbitten hands into hot water. It's remarkable that kids grow up at all, they're so dumb. But that was still a weekend that I'll remember all my life. It was wonderful, and Glenn, with it all, loved "college life."

On February 9, 1972, I walked to Dr. Dube's office. And I sat, waiting. Usually doctors sneak into their offices the back way or through the window or something, but there at the front door, quite late for our appointment, a man with incredible, bushy eyebrows dashed in with his little hat and coat. He was like an animated cartoon, throwing a quick hello toward me and dis-appearing. I am not a patient patient. Also, first appointments are always time-consuming and I was in my usual hurry to get back to my merry-go-round.

To keep me occupied, I was given some kind of application to fill out and, of course, made note of my diabetes. I then voided for a second nurse and read a blurry eye chart.

"I've been having trouble lately reading the charts. I think I need a new prescription."

The doctor then walked in. "Do you know that you have al-bumin in your urine?"

"No," I answered, having forgotten what I'd been told in Miami.

"How have you been doing?"

"OK. I—I've just been having some trouble with my eyes. Things get pretty blurred a lot lately. I need a new prescription. I'm on the tennis team," I now volunteered, sure that that fact insured my basic good health.

"Great," the doctor said with attempted enthusiasm.

He turned off the lights and picked up his ophthalmascope. He looked in one eye and then the other. Then he turned on the overhead light. His voice was quiet, shy and absolutely chilling.

"Son! You've got big troubles."

My heart raced. I mean raced, broke all records. My voice was hysterical.

"What do you mean? I'm an art major. I'm a tennis player. I need my eyes."

He didn't seem to hear me.

"Is your father here?"

"No. That is, he's in the country," I answered wildly as if Marty had just returned from Transylvania or something. Dr. Dube thought I meant he was in the suburbs or on a farm nearby. While I was trying to disentangle myself from all this unbelievable spaghetti, the doctor said, "I'd like to call your parents. May I do that?"

You don't call long distance for a hangnail or even some protein in your urine. I was petrified.

"Yes, of course. You can call my father at his place. His number is . . ."

I really was acting like a robot. Everything was mechanical. I was directed to the outer office, where I gazed out of the window in bewilderment, and then the doctor was standing over me, those eyebrows bristling. No amount of gentleness could make the words he said less than portentous. How sweetly can you tell a boy he is going blind?

"I spoke with your father. He and your mother are taking the first plane. You'll come in with them tomorrow morning."

66

"OK," I answered lightly, my diffidence somehow a denial of tragedy. He could have been asking me for brunch.

"OK," I repeated, somehow knowing deep down that I was no longer in any semblance of control, that I was falling in space and needed my father and mother who loved me and just might save me.

Just two weeks before at the hospital, my eyes had been checked as part of the general endocrinology examination and everything, so they said, was fine. Unless they just blew it and didn't see something. But it was so obvious that this bushy-eye-browed doctor didn't even have to take off his coat and hat and go through a proper how-do-ya-do before he mentioned the word *retinopathy*.

I remember all the terrible things that were said that day at Dr. Dube's. There were no good things. He might not have been diplomatic or psychologically supportive or even very considerate, but, Jesus, he was what I always claim I want from doctors. He was honest.

I do remember mention of some possible treatment, but he'd apparently sprinkled the poisoned facts with just a pinch of false hope. His own apparent distress was touching, his candor, I now see, a compliment. But I didn't want candor. Oh, God, then I wanted to be lied to. Back at the dorm I called my father.

"Dad?"

And the sunny voice briefly gilded the clouds. "Hey. Keep your chin up. Mom and I are flying up tonight."

"Dad. My eyes. He said—"

I was scared shitless and my voice was breaking.

"Gary, now hang in there. It's going to be OK."

"I'm losing my eyes."

"Stop it. And if you are, if the worst comes to the worst, Mom and I will each give you one. One blue, one brown. It'll look odd, but you'll wink a lot."

His laugh was nervous.

"OK, Dad. I'll see you later. OK."

I stood at the window and then I heard someone come into

the room. It was a good friend, Lou Illiano, a guy with whom I was planning a trip to New York City. Something always came up at the last minute to scotch our plans to get to the big town. We were supposed to go that weekend. Lou was a great big guy, warm and funny and six-four. We were a sight gag together— two paces and he could have been home in Flatbush without outside transportation at all.

"Well, looking forward to our trip?" he asked.

"I can't go, Lou."

"Shit! It's always something with you."

"I know, but—"

"What's it this time, pussy?"

"Lou, I think I'm going blind."

"That's original, anyway. The excuses are getting more creative."

I turned around.

"Oh, shit!" my friend moaned.

"Yeah! Look I haven't told anybody yet, and I'd like to live the day as normally as possible. You know, like keep real busy till my parents arrive tonight."

Lou stuck with me and we went out for a good lunch at Haven Hall—which I needed—and then afterward I dropped by the tennis courts and played for a while. I was going through the motions, fighting both failing eyesight and the news that my eyesight was failing. I don't know which was more responsible for my lousy game, but I really couldn't concentrate so I returned to the dorm and brooded. When that proved pointless I called Tom Fairchild and we went to dinner and the Syracuse-Fordham basketball game. We won at the buzzer in double overtime. It was really a great game. Then we went to a little club called the Jabberwocky under Kimmel dining hall to hear Tom Rush. The first song he sang was called "These Days" by my favorite, Jackson Browne.

> I've been out walking,
> I don't do that much talking these days.
> These days I seem to think a lot

                    about the things I forgot to do
                    in all the time I had a chance to . . .
"My God!" I muttered.

I think that no matter the posture we assume, there are times each of us becomes a child again. I know that for all my independence and self-reliance, that night when I went to sleep—knowing that my parents had just arrived and we would all be off to the doctor early in the morning—I was happy to have them in charge, grateful and certain that somehow they would rescue me.

For a split second I was relinquishing all control. When Marge and Marty heard, first hand, the news about my retinopathy, a direct result—indeed one of the prime targets of juvenile diabetes—their reaction was typical. There was no breast-beating and hand-wringing. As emotional as they both are, their first step is always in the right direction. *How can we make this right? What must we do? There is nothing we will not do. Tell us how we can reverse this and make everything right. We will see to it that all will end well. There just is no question about it, all problems in the right hands are soluble.* Amen!

Dr. Dube spoke guardedly about available therapy. There was laser surgery, photocoagulation, and he recommended an ophthalmologist in Syracuse. Step number one. My parents both winked at me affirmatively and we were off only to have the terrible diagnosis confirmed. There was no question. All hell was breaking loose in the retina. Multiple aneurisms were destroying my vision. It was rapidly dwindling.

This was a day for decisions. One two three, I took "temporary" leave from the University in order to go home where, according to Dr. Dube, the University of Miami's Bascom Palmer Ophthalmology clinic was tops. We went to see the Dean in order to arrange for a transfer of credits so I could continue my studies in Miami until I was able to return.

The glare was horrible as I stood looking at Lowe Art School. It was so dazzling that I was temporarily blinded by it. I let my

                                                                    69

father do the rest of the talking while I went back to the dorm to pack. One by one, the guys dribbled in. Starting with one of the tennis captains, Dan Lowengard, each said his good-byes. The news had traveled like the plague.

"Hey, man, I'm sure sorry."

"Will you be coming back?"

"Is there any hope that . . ."

I knew all through the charade about credits that this was it. I knew hope or no hope that I was never coming back. I just knew it, and still I played a game with myself and found something positive about the turn of events. It was insanity, but I remembered that my cousin Janet and our friend Thumper were taking a holiday in Miami at this time and I'd now be able to see them both. It wasn't a fair exchange for my sight, but it was my first down payment on my future sanity. I held on to this thought as if it were a life raft in my sea of trouble. And then my buddy Stacy, who had told me my drawings stank and helped prod me into *trying*, remained as tough as ever as she said good-bye.

"I'll see you later, Stace," I said, adding, "I hope."

She made me ashamed again.

"See to it, Gar."

Her voice was almost threatening in its challenge. Marvelous! Like Slim, like my parents, Stacy wouldn't allow wallowing, and actually it would have bored me.

My roommate, Artie, was terrified that in my desperation I would end the whole business. He didn't really know me. There was too much drama and comedy in the offing. I was too curious about the grisly future.

While Marty and Marge helped me pack, I took a broom Artie and I had. Making it a cane I limped around the room, tapping it on the floor like a metronome before me as I circled the dorm. I made that sweet smile the blind so often sport perhaps to ward away danger. I got my laugh and blurred as my vision was I certainly saw that my audition was killing my parents who had to hear a routine that included, "When I choose a blind date, I'm gonna—like the Yellow Pages—have to let my fingers do the job."

Tom Fairchild, still wearing his ten gallon Stetson said, "When you walk blind, remember, don't walk with your arms straight out in front of you like Frankenstein's thing, because if there's a pole or a tree you'll smack right into it and break your nose. You got to cross your arms first and block anything," and he demonstrated the technique.

And Lou said, "Gary, we got you a going away present—a lot of Jose Feliciano and Stevie Wonder albums."

After a couple of windup Helen Keller stories we had some more laughs. They knew that I would be outrageous to my grave and probably lengthen my exit by getting one last one.

And then sandwiched in between my despair and my need to use it for comedy there was that comforting delusion that somehow my parents would get the doctors to cure me. Certainly an operation, treatments, my own health up to this terrible time would preclude any need for gloom.

In some rosy, distant future, I was going to be whole and tall with twenty-twenty vision and maybe Robin or somebody at my side cheering me on in what looked like my idea of Wimbledon. My family would be in the best seats screaming with laughter as I, brown-legged and sharp-eyed, handily won every set. *This* was the reality. The facts, the delusion.

"Well, guys, I'll be back. They're going to poke my eyes out, clean 'em up and poke them back in again. I'll be seein' ya."

# 9

IT WAS the end of my college career. I did sign up at the University of Miami for some drawing, sculpture and English classes and went immediately to see Dr. Ed Norton at Bascom Palmer. He was out of town and a colleague saw me instead. My condition was diagnosed as papilitis. He believed at that time that it was just a swelling of the optic nerve and he took photographs and discussed odds and percentages as if we were opening a gambling house at Las Vegas. I didn't respond to his detached view of my problems. When I telephoned in desperation while I was hemorrhaging he never answered my calls and when I persisted, he unbelievably told me that he was too busy, and besides there was nothing he could do anyway. He really sounded annoyed.

I will never forget this as long as I live. Surrounded by doctors now for many years, I have scored them as Dudley Moore did his women in "10." There have been plenty of beauties as well as dogs.

Short of a complete and often-times impossible cure, a doctor should give you psychological support and guidance. The collaboration of his treatment and your hopeful acceptance of it is essential. The beginning of any successful treatment is hope of its success. The doctor legitimates this romantic hope with his know-how, his confidence, his honesty and gentle use of all three. There is style, content and common sense.

A warm and emotional doctor in Wisconsin held my hand when I was eighteen, and, in the hushed and consoling tones of a mother at the bedside of her child, informed me that I would be blind in a year and on dialysis or dead in two. She was grief stricken and darling this Dr. Betty Crocker dame as she embroidered the homely sampler, PREPARE YOURSELF FOR YOUR MAKER. If I'd been someone else, I might have fulfilled her prophecy made eleven years ago.

Even when there is a genuine gift, doctors often display a self-protective detachment or overriding ego that denies fallibility. The sick must not only be alerted to their own excesses but those of their healers as well. We must always be on guard. It is no secret that hospitals can be abattoirs, its nurses and medical staff sanctified butchers.

I love life, and as an amateur in the medical field I am dedicated in my pursuit of its extension. I will do my job and simply want no obstacles thrown in my path by professionals. That I bring my own arrogance and sensibility to my own body long afflicted and by this time articulate in its communication with me, is not in the least irrelevant. I am, as many chronically ill are, a specialist without a degree who must be respected and heeded as a consultant. Frankly, I have come to consider most examinations second opinions.

When a doctor's vanity and emotional needs take priority over a patient's well-being, then something must be done. I pity anyone who lands in a hospital with no family or friend to fight for his survival, because exactly this situation is possible. Not too long ago, I experienced this very state of affairs in New York City. It was unreal. Busy, little uniformed bunnies were scampering around in an attempt to administer drugs, which even in my weakened state I knew could prove very damaging. My objections were ignored.

Patients, no matter their intelligence, are often treated like imbeciles by the staff who have rarely been properly briefed as to their individual needs and taboos. If you plead for further consideration you are treated with the same medications plus contempt. One would think that sickness itself was some kind

73

of infraction of divine rules, an affront to the AMA. I may add with great generosity that perhaps it is a stirring and chilling reminder that for all their devoted efforts they, the doctors, are not gods.

Whatever, I suggest that the reader stay healthy and out of their clutches. Having said this, I am alive because of doctors, and as self-appointed guardian, observer and committed preserver of one Gary Kleiman, I am a slouch next to the remarkable Dr. Daniel Mintz, now head of Diabetic Research at the University of Miami Hospital. This gentleman is what a doctor is supposed to be, what medical students dream of becoming and what the sick pray and pay for.

Dr. Mintz has never forgotten that the patient is the reason he is a doctor. The patient when he examines or talks to him is the center of the universe. He is always confident, efficient and feeling. He is never preoccupied—suffering your presence. With Dr. Mintz at your side, even dying would doubtless be the ultimate travel experience. The guy is fantastic.

I once, a long time ago, complained that he was holding out on me, not sharing all his data, and he gently said, "Let me carry my bag of tools. I'll lend you the ones I think you need."

Over the years, Dr. Mintz has let me handle more and more, knowing my need. From the beginning, he would take me to a bar and toast my sugarless soda with his mug of beer. He would ask me questions whose answers were important for me to hear. He helped teach me about myself. Unlike those other doctors, he creates a relationship of mutual respect. He plain old cares.

I know I'm a handful and am presently his sole patient because he is now head of research. He worries about me and feels I take too much responsibility for my own care, but who cares more than I? In reality, I must be my own guardian and hold my own parasol as I walk the high wire. No one, not even he, can equal my dedication to my own survival. I would be lost without the burden, perhaps even unbalanced by it.

His concern, of course, is prompted by compassion. He knows how disheartening it is to show my brand of zeal and discipline and end up exhausted and in exactly the same place I started. Because, so far, status quo is the name of the diabetes game. One has to stay sick. The only alternative—if the complications become too terrible—is not only unavoidable, but preferable.

It will pass, the despair he has detected. He has glimpsed what most have not. He has caught me catching my breath, back in the hospital again after being home, bitter, angry, reeling from still another complication. It will pass. It always does. I'm still around and as long as I am—if I am ever going to show my gratitude to him and others at the hospital—I will continue to beat the lousy odds and be an inspiration to others. But once in a while I'd love to leave the room, take a deep sigh and then resume the performance.

At least I know that *here* in the hospital everything is possible and I can join in my own fight. With all I've said about the medicos, I exclude most happily my surgeon, my nephrologist, my whole incredible gang here. Everything mortally possible is being done for me, but the intangibles loom large and sassy. Cyclosporin is a brand-new drug. Who in hell knows how compatible it is with all the rest of my medications? Trial and error. But it is Dr. Mintz who is even more disappointed than I that at this writing my creatinine reading is still so high. High enough, it reaches autointoxication, uremic poisoning and "So long, folks." He wants so badly for me to come through this, for the drug to be proven, for the decisions made in my treatment to have been judicious, for me to return to my "normalcy." He is my general, he is my friend, and I cannot help but detect the dismay in his voice or the strain in Marty's suddenly haggard face when he visited today.

I really believe that it is worse for those who watch the sick. We are not always brave, but we are onstage and working at it. We are so busy prevailing that we have no time to reflect on the effects. The audience gets the full impact. It is essential that we keep their spirits up, that we control their reactions as best we can. And that goes for the doctors, too.

Daniel Mintz, aside from his own lovely family, has only

wanted two things in the world. To cure diabetes and be a fishing guide. I've been fishing with him without seeing one fish. I have hope. He's got to be good at at least one of them. It was even money, but I'm sure my luck has held.

From the sublime we return to Dr. No, who back in 1972, two weeks after diagnosing me and ignoring my phone calls, saw me before Dr. Norton returned. He now thrilled at the sight of me. Miraculously, it seemed, my eyes had cleared up, the swelling was all gone.

"My God! I'm glad I've documented this. Your eyes are absolutely clear. I can't believe it."

I matched his enthusiasm, wanting desperately to believe it. I would now be able to return to college and other things. I was seeing Robin more seriously and, though she was dating someone else, I threw my hat in the ring. That lovely smile seen clearly again encouraged me.

My drawing classes, especially, or should I say singularly, with Gene Massin were going especially well. He seemed to be the only one who really encouraged me. Because no one was applauding me enough, I was dropping classes right and left, but not Gene Massin's. At Syracuse I was told my drawing was too tight.

"Loosen up, Kleiman."

Here I was being told it was too loose.

"Tighten up, Kleiman."

I decided a plague on both of them.

"I quit," I announced.

But Mr. Massin was different. He talked a lot—about art and life; and his vibrations and huge mustache were great. He was filled with the life juices. I enjoyed his classes immensely and attended diligently.

Things seemed to be improving. Modern science and our own optimism were going to make everything all right. Weren't my eyes OK? And we were building a new and great house and my father's business was booming and so, of course, the phone rang, or rather the bell tolled.

76

An aunt was trying to contact my grandfather, and the next thing we knew my father rushed out of the house to see what was wrong with "Pop," who loved to go bowling with us. With his omnipresent cigar puffing away between his teeth, he would heave the ball and never look up to see if he'd hit a pin. He just loved being with his son and grandsons. It wasn't how you played the game, it was just that you be part of the action.

Two minutes after Marty left, the phone rang again with the news. The old man was dead. I got into my car and tailed my father's to North Miami Beach.

Pop had died in his sleep, and Marty's reaction was something else. I never had seen him like that. He was shattered. His father was dead, and as he looked at me, I read his mind. His son wasn't doing so hot either. Later, at home, it was really heavy. I understood that Pop was great and everything but, after all, I thought, he was *seventy-eight. It's to be expected.* As if the inevitable is necessarily acceptable—or even expectable.

Marty is admittedly an emotional man, but he now held Glenn and me in his arms, crying, "My boys, my boys."

I realized seeing this vibrant man so vulnerable that this grieving son was my father and I could lose *him*, that Glenn and I were sharing for an awesome split second the whole remarkable flow—the continuum. I knew intuitively that this grief was somehow everybody's. Odd! I was out of myself for that second and then I returned to home base. When Marty asked that instead of flowers, donations be sent to the Hope School, a mental institution in Miami, I said, "Why not to diabetes?"

My father's voice was unusually deliberate. "It's going to the *Hope School.*"

One of his sisters had been existing there for years. I had thought of myself and not the daughter of the man who just died. It might have been insensitive, but I still feared—despite my improved vision—that I was going to need a diabetes cure pretty badly. *And* little old me did come first.

I was occasionally driving to classes and otherwise dashing everywhere in my car and with Robin. The eyes weren't perfect, but they were improving. And then one morning as I was walking in the street, I saw a speck in my eye. It floated around and I watched it, fascinated, controlling its travels in reverse by adjusting my gaze. It was a "floater," a harbinger of things to come. This nuisance of a speck trailed every move of my eyes. I couldn't blink it away. It was kind of interesting and I discussed it with Gene Massin, whose *entire* left, walled eye sort of shuffled off to Buffalo. We used to kid about it after I asked where I should concentrate my stare when speaking to him.

On my way to his studio one afternoon, happily driving along, my vision became more and more blurred. It was something like driving through a car wash. I tried insanely to explain it away while my heart pounded, but when I couldn't see whether the traffic light was red or green an alarm went off in my head.

"Shit!" it screamed, "I can kill myself and a lot of other people. I've got to get out of here fast."

And I slowly, practically in slow motion, felt my way back home. *My God,* I thought, *you can't drive. You can't be trusted at a wheel. You're dangerous!*

I got home, parked in front of the house and rushed to my mother's room and fell into a chair near her bed.

"I couldn't see the lights. I can't drive. I couldn't tell whether the lights were green, red, or purple."

I must have been hysterical because my mother who can be operatic in her emotional responses was calm.

"Tomorrow will be a different story. Perhaps tomorrow you'll be able to drive."

I couldn't believe her cool but I did want to believe her. After all, I'd had these dramatic grayouts and then I got better.

This time I did not. I spent a great deal of time at Bascom Palmer and there was no treatment—just new instructions. I mustn't strain myself, not lift anything heavy, sleep with my head elevated. And still my eyes became more and more blurry. It was suggested that I see a Dr. Matthew Davis in Madison, Wisconsin, and Marge and Marty set up an appointment to see him at the university. We all arrived in a blizzard that almost paralyzed the city.

78

The next morning on the way to Dr. Davis's office, we walked down a long hallway lined with people suffering from diabetic retinopathy. Two lines of sitting ducks. I couldn't believe that I was walking into the frame, becoming part of this terrible picture of misery. The endless line of wretches included the elderly, the middle-aged and the young. There was a blind woman in a beige slack suit with a child she had glimpsed only briefly as an infant. One wheelchair had an emaciated legless man with black glasses—diabetes at its most efficient. I remember mostly a sixteen-year-old boy with a white-tipped cane, with everything but a tin cup. Eye patches, crutches, bewilderment were everywhere. Things to come. I could barely contain my anger. It was making my ears feel hot.

These people were all too familiar with the place and each other—like club members—and I knew that if this many people had had these problems for so long, I was in real trouble. It really hit me that I was one of the gang. Sitting between my mother and father, waiting to be examined, I whispered, "You've got to promise that if I become blind, if I ever have to be wheeled to dialysis—" But we were ushered into Dr. Davis's office.

"Your eyes are soaking wet," he said. "I don't know how you can see at all. You should be seeing twenty-two hundred the swelling is so great."

He continued probing. "What else interests you besides art and tennis?" he asked.

"If I'm going to be blind, Doctor, I'd rather be dead."

"But there are alternatives, my boy. Look, we'd like to put you in the hospital for a little while and try some diuretic therapy to relieve your edema."

"But I have tickets for the Rangers in New York, tickets on the blue line. I've never seen a hockey game. While I can still see . . ."

I checked into the hospital immediately and nine million people looked in my eyes. I was Exhibit A. I was given fluorescein—an injection of dye which is then photographed as it travels through the veins. I was a most recent onset case of retinopathy

79

and, since this was also a medical school, I was the medical students' dream. It seems I had galloping retinopathy, which might have been terrible for me but was great for the class. I really felt as if my body had been donated rather prematurely to research. And there was nothing they could do. Galloping or crawling, I wasn't ripe for surgery! There was still no way of treating me.

There was talk of seeing some counselors and I refused. I wanted no pep talks or counseling in how to accept an unacceptable situation. I refused to make this nightmare real. I was furious at everything and everybody. *It isn't fair,* I kept saying to myself. And when I went to the Nielson Tennis Center and watched some games, I almost exploded. I mean, I was really pissed off. *Look at those spastics. They can't even hold a racket but they're playing. They stink and they're hitting the damned ball and I'm good and I can't even find it anymore.* It was like punching the wind, kicking the air, cursing God.

I can't say that the turn of events invigorated or exalted me, but, oddly, it made me more enraged than depressed. I always felt there was hope. I can't live without it. I don't know why or how, but I felt it; and my family, always questioning and searching, was convinced that we would find a way of beating this. Flying home over the clouds and everything—so near to heaven—Marge daydreamed of healthy sons and she prayed.

A retarded child in the adjoining seat, a child she'd been kind to, got airsick and vomited all over her.

# 10

INSTEAD OF IMMEDIATELY returning to Miami with my parents, I insisted on stopping off in Syracuse to say farewell to one part of the future. I had loved Syracuse. I had loved the promise never kept. I may not have honored it at the time, but now something evil had broken it into a million pieces and I had to return to the scene of the crime.

Artie met me and it was the strangest thing. My life had been so compressed, my perspective so foreshortened, that I experienced what Marty had when he'd introduced me to the campus. His disenchantment took twenty years. Mine not much more than twenty weeks. I was no longer part of the school photograph. I was superimposed, the ghost at the banquet—outside looking in. I was starting the aging process that would transform me, like a Hollywood montage, in a matter of seconds. Obscenely out of sync, I flew home to Florida—and just in time.

When I saw Dr. Norton next, and this was just two weeks after Dr. Davis said that I was still untreatable because there was no new vessel growth, I was forced to stay and be treated immediately. It seems as if there had been a jungle growth of new vessels and they had to be destroyed by laser surgery before they affected the healthy ones. But this powerful element is not as selective as one would hope—nor as controllable.

"Which eye are you going to treat, Doctor?"

"We'll have to decide that."

"But my right eye is much worse, so let's bring it back."

"I think, Gary, that the right eye is too far gone."

"Too far gone?"

"I would rather save the left eye."

"Did you say, 'Save the left eye'? I thought we could save everything. I mean, in time, if I do as you say, if—"

I'd spoken dramatically about losing my vision, but I hadn't *really* believed it. We weren't made to believe such things.

Marty had left his business and had come with Marge; they were sitting right outside the office, as they were at all times, through every horror. At school Glenn would be handed bulletins. He was helpless. My mother and father questioned Dr. Norton as if they were grading him on some lofty examination. He passed all right—with flying colors. We have never lost our respect for him. He was not just an eye doctor. He understood everything he saw in a patient's eyes—but everything. My parents examine all possibilities and aren't intimidated by the white coats. They decided to trust his judgment and we three, after discussion, agreed to laser my *left* eye.

I was given Valium intravenously and I got a real high on. Easily affected by all medications, I was smashed.

"Hey, where did you get this stuff? Does the fuzz know? My buddies at college would go ape."

We all started to laugh and the tension was broken. Dr. Norton now gave me a retrobulbar injection, one directly underneath the eye and I felt severe pressure but no pain. A dazzling light now blazed, burned and bored through my skull. Only a weird sensation in the back of my head accompanied the glare. Contrary to everything I've ever heard about relative time, I thought I was there for about ten minutes and it turned out to be an hour. Along with the drug and my own agitation, time was obviously shortened by the mystery and horror of this, my first xenon photocoagulation, one form of laser surgery that destroys the wild and woolly cells or vessels that hemorrhage and eventually affect the healthy ones causing blindness.

82

I was still an amateur doctor in those days and I am grateful that Dr. Norton wisely worked on the left eye instead of the right which was being destroyed by aneurisms and new, wild vessels and was, indeed, too far gone to have been cured. What I could see I perceived through veils of blood—not red (and this could not be seen by anyone looking at me)—but black ink that moved in waves and tides like a fishbowl tipped one way and then the other. If I just sat still and stared it was like a Rorschach test. I could play "what is it?" for hours as the slightest motion changed the awful eyescape. When the patch was removed from the treated eye, there was, I told Dr. Norton, "total blackness."

"Impossible. There must be something, *some* vision," the doctor insisted.

"No, just a speck of light in the lower left-hand corner."

"Ah, that's different."

"Different?" I repeated. "It might just as well be total. *I can't see.*"

"But you should," Dr. Norton said. "When the eye is no longer traumatized. The healthy vessels will recover now. Believe me."

"I would rather be dead," I repeated.

Speck of light and promises notwithstanding, it was now suggested that I meet with someone from the Bureau of Blind Services. Against my will, a woman came to the house and slobbered over me, after which she asked how my hearing was and if I would come and have my ears examined. Her unwelcome presence, her ready acceptance of my fate and this nonsense about my ears unbalanced me.

"It's my goddamned eyes, you idiot!" I bellowed, running out of the house, where I sulked beneath a sea grape tree until she left.

Marty gave me holy hell. "I know you're angry and you're right to be angry. But you don't have to be unkind and rude to anyone."

It seemed to me at the time that two gentlemen in the family were enough.

I was lashing out all over the place. In a month I was seeing virtually nothing. I remember some friends of Glenn's coming over to visit and sitting on his bed and having a bull session. I couldn't make out one face. And one night I didn't recognize my own mother crossing the room. Things were getting darker and darker and I wrote Robin an eleven-page letter discouraging any further relationship—on *any* level, which was a presumption since I wasn't in control of that situation either. She could now see someone who was healthy and, in an attempt to deprive myself of everything worthwhile, I said my farewells. It was all very dramatic and self-sacrificing.

"What is this crap?" she asked when she received the tome.

I adored her.

"What is this crap?"

We became inseparable. She helped me train my puppy shepherd, Dylan, and encouraged me, laughed with me and with time-honored teen-age sentiment made me listen carefully to Bill Wither's new song, "Lean on Me." It was to be our song. *My God*, I thought. *Our Song. I'm having a romance. I'm a boyfriend.* Dylan wasn't the only puppy, but I craved Robin and our affection saved my sanity.

It isn't sensible to evaluate by current detachment the depth of my feeling. At that time I was in love. It's fascinating, sitting here and smiling tolerantly over my immaturity ten years ago, but those feelings were real and I must honor them. I was learning to feel, and if my lessons were to be wasted like youth on the young, so be it, or in our case, so it was.

I so hungered for Robin's company and affections that one evening when she couldn't come because the family car was not at her disposal, I was distraught. No one was at home at my place to give me a lift and, of course, I was no longer driving. Robin lived a mile and a half away. I started at dusk and felt my way along the roadways and streets by shadow. When I arrived at her driveway, it was dark and I saw nothing. I remembered Tom Fairchild's advice and crossed my arms before my eyes and managed to get to her front door free of accident but totally drained. I was soaking wet when she answered the bell. She couldn't believe that I had done this on my own. But I had to see her, had to move when I wanted to and had to be on my own.

That night we shared the dark and heavy things. The sudden death of her father a short time before, the senseless loss of her baby sister, run over by a hit-and-run driver right at their front door. Two people she loved snatched from her. She knew what it was to feel strongly and she cried softly as she spoke of these things. There was no doubt that she was feeling my pain too and now I felt hers.

"Why are you crying?" she asked angrily. But we'd touched each other. At least I had this speck of light.

In June they tried another type of laser treatment called Argon. This time my head was strapped to a machine while drops were administered. Then a contact lens that looked like a mini-telescope was poked into my eyeball and a laser beam was shot into the very center of my head. I could feel it ticking and click-ing. There were hundreds of zaps, zapping, rat-a-tatting like a sta-pler. My family was sitting outside the office and Glenn was with them. Every time he heard the zap, which vibrated through the wall, he beat his fist against it. Our parents had two boys to com-fort.

# 11

I've been back at the damned hospital for the last few days with a virus as well as other complications. Now a virus is never a welcome guest. It's more like a party crasher. In my case, it is a marauder and quite possibly a killer. I have enough trouble with the invited outsiders with names like Cyclosporin and Medrol and Lasix—I could go on forever. My body is always having open house.

"If I had the wings of an angel!"

The sun is shining through the window; the sky is blue-blue and in my fatigue and disgust a scene from my childhood flashes across the darkness of my eyes.

The urge to flee somewhere has made me recall that day when I was five years old and up to my neck with the restrictions placed upon my hyperactivities. My mother's rules and regulations had driven me to extreme measures. I would be free. I stole several garbage bags from the kitchen and went to my room where Marge was tidying up a mess I had made and had been punished for. I solemnly filled the bags with my toys as I prepared to leave home.

"Well," Marge said with satisfaction, "you've decided to clean up and act like a real person. That's a good boy."

"I'm not cleaning up; I'm not a good boy."

"What are you doing?"

"I'm leaving."

I ran around the room collecting trucks, toy soldiers, blocks, planes and animals as my mother sat on the edge of the bed and watched me.

"You mean you're running away? Leaving home?"

"Yes."

The garbage bags were soon filled to brimming and I was ready to depart. I knew she would beg me to stay, make any concession, that any second she would burst into tears. I was determined to leave anyway. I'd had enough.

"Are you finished packing?" Marge asked.

"Yes."

"Don't you think you might like to take some clothes, a toothbrush, some food in case you get hungry?"

I was mortified. I hadn't thought of these things. She was acting *so* grown up.

"I won't need them," I said loftily, imitating her tone.

"Then it's good-bye," Marge said.

I left—barely able to lug those dead weights behind me. Sheer will got me to the street, but since I wouldn't jettison even one of my precious possessions and fearing that I would lose everything, I returned unchastened but quick to grab the cake and milk awaiting me in the kitchen. I accepted them as an apology. That was before cake was poison or medicine, but just a pleasure.

Healthy children are like animals or flowers. They just are. For a while there it's all so simple. Of course, disease afflicts all things and even the elements can ravage a dainty life. But the tree, though stationary, is free to reach for the sky, the colt to race for its prized horizon. They don't consider the mechanics. Whatever their limitations or expectations, they were built in millions of years ago. After all this time, I envy them, not for myself, I don't think, but for my kids, who will one day share my predicament, unless! Diabetes-stricken children have ahead of them a lifetime of tyranny if they aren't educated to responsibility and self-rule and then—on top of it—it's a matter of luck. They must be lucky.

Even now, I am fighting my years-long battle at the hospital.

Out again, in again. I knew one of the new medications was wrong for me. I felt it. With no proof except for my turning worse after its prescription. They are looking for the ideal formula and I must be patient and grateful. We're all guessing at this point. Their guesses are educated, my hunches inspired. They've got to be the bosses right now, but the stakes are awfully high.

One more trip to Madison, Wisconsin, proved fruitless. It was suggested there that I have a pituitary operation, an idea which we happily rejected. On returning to Miami Beach, I just hung around the house in depression.

I was anything but heroic. I wavered between self-pity and towering rage. I'd received so many mixed messages from so many different sources that I could pay my money and make my choice but the general mood was black. I couldn't sit and stare so I just sat. Dr. Norton had told my family to allow me a period of mourning.

"He has lost his vision and he must grieve. Let him allow the sighted boy to die."

And I did. I became a zombie between rages. I sputtered and flared at almost anything and my impatience, bitterness and short fuse set the mood for the entire household. There is no describing my frustration. I had always been the safari guide but now I was cannibal as well and chewed everyone's head off. I have never been a saint and don't understand the incredible humility that allows for such benign acceptance of the Devil's will. There just didn't seem any way to fight back. I would have. I just gritted my teeth, clenched my fists but I couldn't beat the shit out of diabetes or land even one good left jab at You Know Who!

Marge and Marty wept together. They continued to do everything together. First of all, it was their way, but back in Miami while I was making that return visit to Syracuse they went on Lois Meitus's advice to see a Dr. Lipton, a psychiatrist. On the way to his office, they saw a man selling pencils in Coconut Grove and they almost went mad.

Dr. Lipton told them that he couldn't console them, that

some things were only consolable in time. He said that he couldn't lighten their burden or take their pain away, but that the most positive thing they could do was to face the horror squarely, not to shut each other out, not to try unburdening the other, but to suffer *together*. How great. How remarkable that this man understood that need.

"Though it gnaws at you, though the tension makes you fractious, though your individual reactions can tear at you, your common pain will make you closer. Share everything. He's *your* son."

And so they suffered and they even suffered me together. Now with everything else I had the jitters. I would go through the ceiling like Halley's comet in a hurry to make my black and blue streak. My God, what all this did to everyone. And Marge and Marty never gave up.

I saw things differently out of the pinpoint of vision I had in that traumatized left eye. Only a miracle could save me, but that's exactly what Dr. Meitus offered as a possibility if I went to Duke University to one Dr. Kempner whose rice diet was controversial but had some highly publicized success with retinopathy as well as hypertension. We preferred to concentrate on the successes and not the disappointments.

Of all the periods of subjugation I've endured, there was none so terrible to me as the Rice House at Duke University in Durham, North Carolina, where tobacco is king killer and everything almost went up in smoke.

The "Rice House" was, among other things, a spa for people with too many pounds and enough dollars to make an attractive exchange. Celebrities paid a bloody fortune to be starved in the seamiest surroundings imaginable. But the beauty part was the possible reversal of my diminishing sight.

There was nowhere else to turn at this point and Marge and Marty decided to pack our bags in the blind hope that Durham would become—as it apparently had to others—Lourdes. My grandparents were recruited to watch over Glenn who was in high school. As always they generously pitched in.

He suffered silently, resigning himself to the necessary decision, as usual making certain by his calm and acceptance that he would in no way add further anguish to our frantic parents. What a terrible fate—to be compelled not to make waves. One can drown that way.

In a few short months everything I loved was being threatened. My art, my tennis and my Robin. She came to say good-bye and cried. I wasn't sure why. That ambiguity had remained to torment me, discouraging a full commitment. I couldn't be sure how she really felt. I only knew that I needed her devotion and knew I would have to spurn it. Oddly, too patly, the radio was playing "In My Mind I'm Going to Carolina" and then, incredibly, our "Lean on Me." I remember praying that, if the worst happened and I became totally blind, I would retain the image of her lovely face forever. In just a few months one shock after another had forced me to admit to my friend Thumper that "they can't seem to fix me. I may never see again."

I heard her voice shake as she said, "Oh, God!"

"Yeah," I'd answered.

I insisted that Robin drive my car while I was away and promised to write and call every day. I had no idea I'd be at Duke for nine months.

# 12

**W**ITHOUT AN OFFICIAL appointment with the great
doctor, I had to go through a preliminary screening
that made matriculation at Heidelburg or Oxford—
not to mention Syracuse—child's play. The tests were endless
and failing them insured your acceptance. And then the professor
appeared. Herr Doktor, Walter Kempner in person, no facsimile.

I am sure that Dr. Kempner clicked his heels in his sleep. I
was even surer that he ran the "Rice House"—which my family
called "The Last Chance Cafe"—like occupied territory. Typically Prussian, Dr. Kempner was lean, redoubtable and utterly au-
thoritarian. He usually wore a blue blazer and sported a gold
stethoscope. The rates were high at the Rice House. I found him
truly bizarre. He didn't have the foggiest idea that his crazy
accent transformed his most serious pronouncements into low
comedy.

"So yor de boi!"

He now raised three fingers.

"How many?"

"Three," I answered.

"Gut! Very gut! You should send your doctor diamonds for
sending you to me."

He was as sure of himself as I'd always been. *Gut!* I thought. *I
love real pros.*

"By the time you leave here, you will be fine," he now announced.

It was the first positive thing we'd heard in months, and a thrill went through me. I was starved for good news in any language. *I'm going to be fine, he said. I won't be blind.*

"But you must do *exactly* as I say."

I knew by just looking at him that that was going to be the price but to be fine I was willing to pay it and double. On his office wall were rows of pictures. Before and after pictures of his grateful patients. He loved them. Before and after! Tubs of lard that had become, with his rice diet, sticks of butter.

"You stay on my diet and you vill be fine. De rice vill kure you. You vill eat rice und fruit and then fruit und rice. And you vill be vell."

"I'll eat bullshit if you'll help my eyes, Doctor."

"Dis I've never hurd, never. Vallpaper, yah!"

"Wallpaper, too, Doctor. Yah to everything—only help me."

I was under his spell. I was going to stand at attention everytime he said *Achtung.* He was going to save my eyes.

"You vill be vell if you do exactly as I say," he now repeated slowly.

I was convinced.

"*If* you do *not*—"

His voice trailed off ominously.

"If you leave before I say—"

His look pierced my gut. The implications were clear. And so the groundwork of fear was laid. I was to feel captive for months. But that was OK. There was hope now.

Marge, Marty and I now took a good look around. The doctor wanted me to live on the premises but we found it depressing. The Rice House was a dingy, tacky, soon to be condemned, three story house with loose floor boards, creaky doors, and it had obviously been decorated by a patient with advanced retinopathy. Early ugly! This was the main building. There was another equally inviting.

Marge shot a glance at Marty who shot a glance at me who now looked back at my mother. Her head was glass. She had two choices. One was to repair, repaint and redecorate and Two was to move us into a nearby hotel until she could find more civilized lodgings. In the months ahead there were several such places that filled the bill with increasing adequacy.

That first dinner in the dining room where I took all my meals is unforgettable. It was like walking into a Botero canvas. I never saw so many fat people in my life. And I'm talking fat. Individuals, not groups, weighed five and six hundred pounds. Some, it was said, even more. They were whales.

I was there, now doomed to this terrible, saltless diet of rice on rice on rice with enough fruit to keep me from getting beri beri, because I was saving my eyesight and kidneys. Many of these patients were actually on summer vacation, greedily starving themselves to be beautiful. It was like a club to the affluent who came there to lose weight only to go home and stuff themselves again.

Some of these people, often celebrated, were regulars who like unregenerate criminals paroled, landed back here periodically. Persons with no willpower and no self-esteem. And *they* were the healthy ones. The rest of us were not there for cosmetic reasons but grave medical ones. Still, the loss of weight improved everyone's appearance as well as ailments. Except for me. I went there in June at one hundred and thirty pounds and kept losing. They could have slipped me under the doctor's door every morning. An "after" picture of me looked like a snapshot taken in a concentration camp, which brings us back to the regimen.

Every morning there was a weigh-in and blood pressure checks before our breakfast of rice and then there was a long walk. Exercise was extremely important. Then there was lunch of rice and more walking. There was about eight miles a day and no intelligent talk. Just gab about fat and thin, before and after, followed by dinner—of rice. For variety we had a choice of cream of rice or white rice. And as a special treat, puffed rice. Talk about running the gamut. One of the first days a girl at my table watched me picking at the fruit cocktail and staring at the mound of dry rice.

"No, no. That's not the way to do it. You'll never get your dinner down that way."

"What are you talking about?"

"You make a hole in the hot rice," she instructed, "and then you pour the fruit into it. It's the only way it's edible."

This was not *cordon bleu*. The first time I tried for some variety and ordered puffed rice, it was so dry that my deep sigh blew it all over the dining room.

Marty, who could have been in worse shape, decided—I wonder why—to go on the diet with me: He claimed he was curious. From the beginning he and Marge spelled each other in Durham, very rarely leaving me on my own, despite my protests. I did send for Dylan, my dog, however, and he remained my one joy. His congenial company, his slimness and his real sympathy for my plight heartened me. My sight was so bad that I kept tripping over him. He accepted everything as long as I turned on the television set in my room. He was addicted to it.

This intelligent animal would become a tail-wagging, paw-twitching simpleton seemingly mesmerized by variety and talk shows, soaps, anything. He was especially fond of the evening news. He was also the only one I was even polite to. My parents suffered my rages more than anyone. I just couldn't be civil to them. They were the closest and those to whom with my medical needs I was most beholden. Why wouldn't they get the worst of it?

I had by this time become a young curmudgeon. What a shit I was! I hated the Fates who sent me to such place and I hated myself for somehow earning their hatred. I was losing both my sight and my mind and there was little I could do but follow the rules. My fellow inmates conspired with each other to cheat on the diet. I don't know who they thought they were fooling. I became a zealot. I would follow *Herr* Kempner to Valhalla if necessary. And when I was dead of boredom, not a trace of salt would be found when I reached that last void.

Of course, aside from the strictness of the diet, I continued my shots of insulin. After all, I was still diabetic. That fact couldn't be lost in the more dramatic results of it. That was the rock in the snowball. I was going to be a good boy and I was going to get out of this joint alive and "vell." But I had to run an obstacle course.

It wasn't hard at nineteen to be everybody's sex symbol at the Rice House. When I took my daily and prescribed walk, my lope turned into a gallop as I fled the stampede of elephants on my tail. It was grotesque. I must have been the only young person there without a weight problem. Hence, I was the house beauty. I was made to feel among these mammoth creatures like the only girl on a pirate ship.

One of my admirers was a girl I'll call Bertha. There aren't words large enough to describe her. She was a compulsive eater and managed to sit at my table whenever she could manage it. One night while Marty was there, she joined us, her soft, wet eyes melting further at the sight of me and the steaming plate of rice set before us. Marty, with no medical problem, was allowed on occasion to have some "real food" and this night had some chicken on his plate. When he was finished Bertha looked around the dining room furtively to see if Herr Doktor was about. Satisfied that he was not, she then—in the swiftest of gestures—grabbed all of Marty's chicken bones in her fat fist and stuffed them in her mouth, oohing and ahing, her eyes rolling as she sucked them dry.

But everybody was obsessive.

"How are you, Mrs. Guggleheimer?" someone would ask.

"Two pounds, Mr. Gallagher," she would answer in triumph.

"Is it a nice day?"

"*Nine pounds*, I swear."

"You should have seen me *before*."

"You mean this is *after*?"

"I can get into the green dress again."

"I can get into trouble again."

I thought I'd go mad. One day when Dylan on lead stopped to sniff a miniature poodle with a diamond collar, the Kaiser happened to pass. The two dogs were so disparate in size, so obviously incompatible for the plans they were making that I had to laugh. Kempner took fleeting note of the scene from his vantage point.

"Before and After," he muttered as he marched by.

When I'd first arrived, Kempner had attempted a light, bantering style.

"Well, jung mann, you are nice looking boy. Perhaps you meet some nice girl and have romance."

"You're kidding, Dr. Kempner. I'm not *that* blind. I've cased the joint. But *nothing*. There are no women here only mammals."

"Vait, mein freund, after a couple of months anything vill look good to you. You'll see. De vorst one vill look gorgeous."

I guess we are all different. With what's left of my eye for beauty I could never be that desperate. It would have been like sinking into quicksand, never to be heard from again. I lived a monk's life at Durham for nine months but I managed to weave a few pleasant dreams into the general nightmare.

I wrote and called Robin daily as I'd promised. After I was there about a month she came for a visit and stayed with us in our apartment. This was a tonic. I was able to share the horror with her and she saw first hand what she hadn't believed. These mastadons proudly opening their shirts and bodices to reveal their sagging flesh.

We laughed and talked and when she left I promised I would try to come home for an Eric Andersen concert. It would be just a weekend and I needed the respite. I would, of course, continue my diet. After all one can eat rice anywhere—even in China—and this was just forty-eight hours in Florida. Well, Kempner went into a rage. He stormed off and got my parents. He then picked up the aria where he'd left off.

"There are plenty doctors from here to Boston. Go. But if

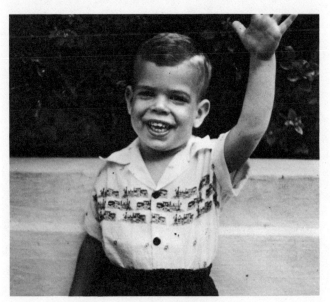

Hi, world!

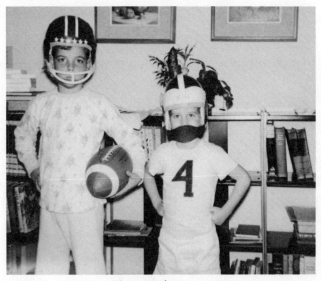

The start of a team

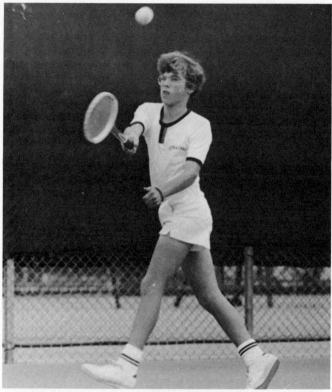

B.C. (Before Complications)

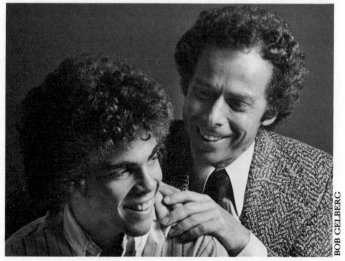

With my father, A.D. (After Diabetes really starts)

BOB GELBERG

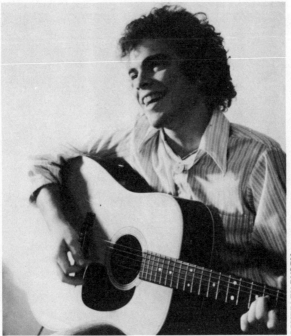

Escaped into music

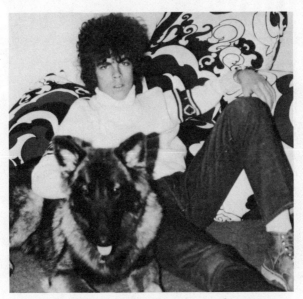

But Dylan was the only one I was polite to

SCHIERLEY BUSCH

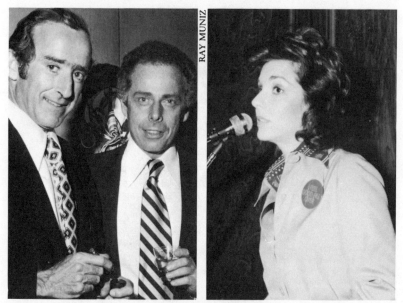

Dr. Mintz and my father        Mother unwillingly becomes a speaker

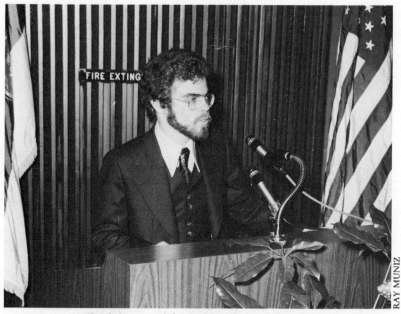

The dedication of the Diabetes Research Institute

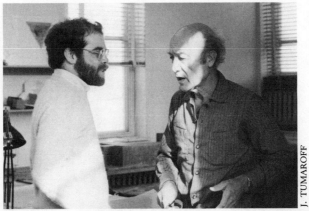

With Isamu Noguchi

J. TUMAROFF

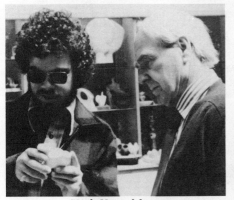

With Henry Moore

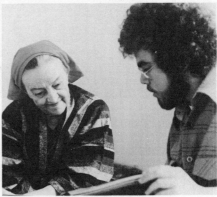

With Barbara Hepworth

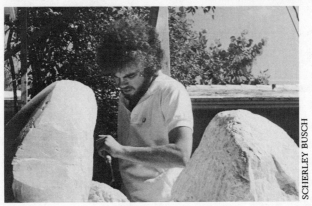

On my own

SCHERLEY BUSCH

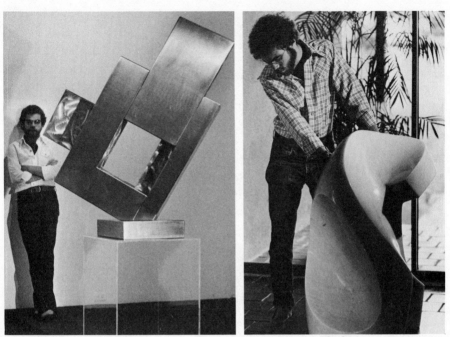

Puzzled

The horse

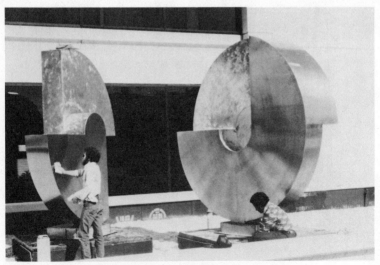

Installation of positive-negative at Bascom Palmer

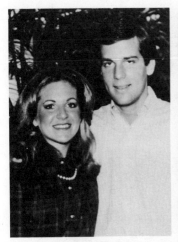

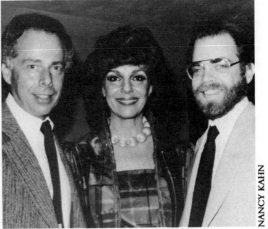

Gise and Glenn

Three fourths of the team

NANCY KAHN

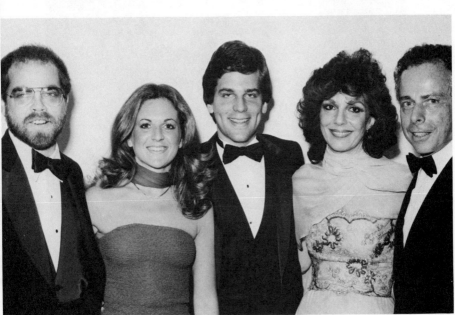

The whole team

RAY MUNIZ

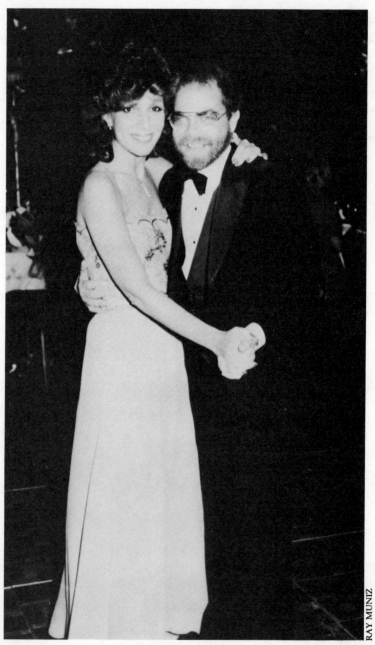

A promise kept

RAY MUNIZ

you go you never come back. You hear? If you vant this boi cured, you *stay*. If you leave—Vell!"

The silence was so foreboding that Marge shivered and Marty assured him that I would stay.

On one trip back home my father had fainted in our bathroom from saline depletion and our other dog, Star, had awakened him by licking his face. Quite unreasonably they now felt that a premature departure from the master would have me withering and dying. We were petrified. He had built up this invincibility, this indispensibility, this thing. We actually believed that without him I was doomed. He was a human Iron Lung or dialysis machine. No Kempner, no life. I felt I was going to have to be there the rest of my life.

In fairness, the blasted diet worked the first weeks. There was immediate benefit. My eyes were better, the right one less filled with edema, the left extending its vision ever so slightly toward the center as Dr. Norton had said it could. I was so impressed with the initial improvement that I wrote to Dr. Davis in Wisconsin impulsively.

"I'm writing this by hand to prove that I can see. I think you should send other people here for the rice diet. It has certainly helped me." And it had, but I was somewhat hasty in my testimonial.

My parents assured Dr. Kempner that I was going nowhere when he made that scene about the weekend junket and we settled down again. *You'd better prove it, Mister,* I thought. *You said that I'd be well again. I'm staying but it'd better pay off.*

I got thinner and thinner until I almost disappeared. I was so emaciated that they had to supplement my diet with spaghetti. All the Ricers agreed that all that was left of me was an afro, green eyes and tennis shoes. But I was more attractive than ever. The spaghetti on my plate was catnip.

"Is that *spaghetti?*" the gourmets would scream as they connived to filch it. Incredible!

Marty, much too thin, himself, had to return to his thriving but neglected business. Fortunately my mother's brother Bill kept it going until my father headed home. He was certainly healthy but he looked changed to me. Not as young, kind of bleached out. For me there was no exit for a while.

# 13

TIME CRAWLED BY. And I became more and more insufferable. Buddy Hackett, the comic, showed up for his annual, halfhearted battle with obesity and made sure his presence was known. He seemed driven, pathetically eager to be funny, and I wasn't in the mood to be amused or singled out for anything by these people in this place in this wretched mood.

"Look at the skinny kid!" he squealed the first day he arrived. I was one hundred and twelve pounds at that point, the birth weight of some of my housemates.

"Look at him! What are *you* doing here?"

The spot was on me now, and I always cringe at my answer.

"You're so fat, I certainly know what *you're* doing here."

Any charm I had ever had I'd neglected to bring to the whole Duke University scene. I was hateful. Mr. Hackett, whatever his needs, was certainly more socially acceptable than I was and he was much kinder. One day in his studied joviality he was showing a snapshot of his kid to one of the fat ladies. She handed it to me enthusiastically and, of course, it was pointless.

"What's the matter, kid? Aren't you interested?" he asked.

"It's my eyes. Diabetes . . ."

And his reaction was real.

"Listen here, kid. I've seen great things here. I mean, you just keep trying and great things will happen."

He was genuinely touched, inviting me and my "girlfriend"

to his hotel for drinks and laughs. He was kind but I fear not prophetic. My period of grace was short and the right eye worsened as what was left of the lasered left seemed slowly to recover. My mood kept darkening and I became even more sullen. I ignored everyone. My father on his many stays listened to everybody's problems. With all that was happening, with all his preoccupation, he always had time for everybody who needed an ear or a shoulder.

"How can you spend so much time with *them*," I would ask in disbelief.

"Because they need someone. Because they're depressed."

"They're depressed because they're fat and won't get a hold of themselves."

I had, I'm afraid, no respect for the kind of sickness that created its own problems. Once affected, these chubbies then did little or nothing to cure themselves. They all wanted instant cures with no disciplines. In their gluttony they all seemed to want what no one in this life ever gets—a free lunch. I had nothing but contempt for their refusal to help themselves. It never occurred to me that some of them couldn't. It was this very lack that made Marty feel for them.

I wouldn't, couldn't understand. The charm and energy he expended on those people! Treating them like Hollywood starlets. I would see them during the day on one of the hikes and I'd quickly turn tail. I had mean and terrible nicknames for them; and my father would walk among them like a priest making a benediction.

One girl for whatever kinky reason kept sending me pictures of Sophia Loren and Raquel Welch, perhaps hoping that I might think they were pictures of her, although that doesn't make sense. Another sent me candles, perhaps to burn down the place with. I'm not as naive as I was then. Their motivations have become too obscene to contemplate. Anyway, I was rejecting everything and everybody and played so much gin rummy with the family that I became drunk on it.

With a new and pleasanter apartment, I decided on a project.

I redid the joint exactly as I had my dorm in Syracuse. It was the beginning of my own therapy. The overture. Because after that, when one young woman gave me a nice picture she had snapped of me and Dylan, I decided to do a sketch of it for my mother's birthday.

It turned out to be the last thing I did with my right eye. I had returned to art; and the picture of Dylan and me walking through the university gardens so pleased me that I told Dad that I was going to bring it home personally. I'd already asked the formidable doktor and he'd agreed that I could go for the weekend. I had been there for months now and he must have felt I would have blown up but for this release.

"Dad, I'm coming home for Mom's birthday. It's all settled. Kempner says OK and I want to surprise her, so mum's the word."

"I've never kept a secret from your mother."

"Dad! This is different. It's a good secret. You're not doing a bad thing. Promise you won't say a word."

"OK. OK. But—"

I wouldn't allow for buts. Unbelievably, Kempner was allowing me this short parole and I wanted to see Marge's face. The whole plan was that I frame the large charcoal and hang it in my bedroom and have my mother come in and say, "What is this?" and I would jump out of the closet and say, "How do you like it?" and "Happy Birthday," and for a change there'd be some warm, great vibes instead of all the shit we'd been through.

Dad and I flew home and everything went as planned. I heard her coming and my heart was beating really fast and there was the picture hanging on the wall looking great and Marge who misses nothing and would notice a new scratch on a windowpane shouted, "Marty! Who did that? Who did that?" And her voice was shaking and Jack in the Box shouted, "How do you like it? Happy Birthday," and my mother almost died. I mean, really almost cooled.

She couldn't stop sobbing and almost collapsed. It turned out to be the most awful thing that I did. I mean, it was really terrible because I guess my mother isn't the person to surprise. She could evidently handle shock but not surprise. It all ended happily but it wasn't the thing to do.

I then decided to repeat the whole business with Robin. I manufactured a book and on each page I wrote one word. "Dear—page—Robin—page—I—wanted—to—come—down—to—surprise—you" and while she was reading it I slowly walked into the room and watched her turning the pages. The book ended with, "I—wanted—to—surprise—you—and—I—did." And Robin shouted, "And so you did?" And I whispered (I was so close to her), "So I did."

This one really worked well. She really flipped and we had a great weekend together. The greatest. And then I had to go back. But it was the turning point. That taste of freedom did it.

On my return my left eye was no longer blistering but my right was hemorrhaging more and more. Concerned, Kempner asked, "Vy don't you hov your girl freund come up and go to school here?" He thought that he'd better find more creative ways of keeping me there since I was now losing faith in his cuisine and he felt he needed more time.

Winter had arrived and with it a whole new set of inmates. I was as resistant as ever but met a remarkable fellow. His name was Meredith. We called him Flash since he had been an Olympic track star. He was presently a physicist—a Cornell man. He was brilliant, black and great in every way. Totally blind from diabetes, he never stopped his regimen of exercise, diet and medications. He couldn't have been more positive in his approach to everything. He couldn't quite revive my spirits but he tried.

As a result of my letter to Dr. Davis, he sent to Durham to join our merry group a young diabetic girl of seventeen who was hopelessly ill. Jan simply sat and her parents cared for her as if she were a sick doll. I mean she did nothing for herself. Her arms and legs were slack like a marionette's.

Her apparent surrender to her destiny touched me and for the first time at Durham I cared about someone else. I was becoming a fixture at the place and as a veteran I would be asked for advice, which I loved giving. I really felt sympathy for Jan, particularly, and another blind fellow who became friends and a kind of responsibility. They had been victimized by sickness, not gluttony. I shared their concerns and was somewhat diverted from my own.

Still, the only person at the Rice House I admired and looked up to was Flash. He was really strong in misery, impatient with me or anyone who for a moment curled up with self-pity or bitterness, which is really the same. I couldn't afford more of that. Flash was overcoming, and no matter what, he was still going to be black and brilliant and therefore doubly handicapped. He was the greatest.

I now decided that I was going to be stronger than anyone. Not bossy, but strong. I was going to be tough as nails and I was going to lick anything. Except you-know-who's boots. My eyes were now getting worse. I clenched my jaw as I started plunging into the deepest of depressions.

I had lived to see in the year 1973 with Robin on the beach back home. It was the first time I'd beaten the odds and proven that lady doctor's prophesy crap. It was a triumph, and when a few charmers at the Rice House asked, as my college roommates had, if I were contemplating suicide, I realized that I had never under *any* apprehension or direst of anticipations even remotely considered it. The life force is strong in me, strongest when it's being most threatened. What a question.

"Dr. Kempner," I attacked, "how can you say I'll play tennis and paint? How can you when I'm gushing blood again in my right eye. You promised I'd be OK."

Loving music I'd bought many records and many tapes when I was at Duke. I played them all day and night but there was no record as persistently replayed as his, "If you stay on your diet, you vill play tennis, you vill draw, you vill drive again." It was a broken record.

"How can you repeat that after all these months? I've done everything you've asked and more! And I'm getting worse. If I have to eat one more bowl of that shit . . . my sodium count has been under ten every single day. I have never cheated. I don't have one damned grain of salt in my urine. *I'm not getting better!*"

"You must be patient!"

"Patient? I've been here practically one nineteenth of my life," I shouted, displaying an uncharacteristic grasp of mathematics.

My strict adherence to the damned diet was not a fiction. I was too scared to break it. I had too much to lose. It had obviously worked for many others but, after that initial benefit, not for me. Still, I was, I felt, in bondage. As for Kempner, I really could run out of metaphors. But not quite. I haven't used the most obvious. To me he was a Teuton Svengali and we were all—everybody there in the Rice House—under his spell. I had to break that spell.

I hadn't thought of myself as one of his subjects until it was time to make my getaway but now I was nervous. Still, I had to be free.

I knew intuitively that whatever disciplines I had learned there, whatever improvement in my condition, there was no longer any possibility of a cure and no fault of his. God knows he tried. I just knew it was over, that it wasn't going to be OK and all the spiel was nothing but strudel in the sky.

It was just at this point that Marge called from back home. Janet Chusmir of the *Miami Herald* wanted to do a story about me in order to help raise funds for diabetic research. The idea excited her and me. What I had experienced personally, in Madison and Duke and in Dr. Norton's office convinced me that for others and myself, the only answer was to prevent or cure diabetes before it ravaged. I was almost twenty but it was obvious that if I was ever to see better days, I was never going to see them clearly and perhaps—and that was my greatest terror—I might not see them at all.

# 14

**M**Y YOUTH WAS OVER, most of my vision irreversibly gone and my prognosis equally murky. I had seen the promise of diabetes kept with a vengeance. Once begun, the erosion caused by this disease was unstoppable. Life-saving as insulin is, it doesn't always save your limbs, your eyes or organs. Marge was right. Although I personally would initially recoil from such exposure, a frank interview could alert others to the wickedness in such delusion.

Mrs. Chusmir conducted the interview by telephone during my last days at Durham and the piece made quite a splash in the Miami *Herald.* It was a strange experience for me, airing so personal an experience, but in a way it made it easier having all the facts out in the open. People were usually so roundabout in their dealings with my illness. Now, astonishingly enough, I was grinning out of the newspaper at people's breakfast tables, confiding to them, not asking for pity, but money for the research that our doctors had once told us was necessary.

The stars really must have been in conjunction or something because there was now a remarkable confluence of events. President Nixon was decreasing federal aid programs and had just reduced by forty-two million dollars the research appropriations of the National Institute of Health, the government's main source of cash for biomedical research.

Dr. Daniel Mintz, at the University of Miami School of Medicine was then investigating the feasibility of implanting insulin producing cells of the pancreas and had been granted an extension of funds now so abruptly withdrawn.

Coincidentally, just prior to my return from the hell-hole at Durham, a family friend, Arthur Kline, became executor of an estate and suddenly had at his disposal ten thousand dollars which at his discretion he could donate to any worthy cause. Arthur and Sheila were old friends and aware of both my condition and my parents' desperate search for help, he asked if they had any suggestions.

"How about Dr. Kempner?" Marge and Marty asked me.

"How about no way," I answered.

The next day, Marge bumped into an old acquaintance in a parking lot—Florence Rubin—who also had a child with diabetes. Along with several other like couples, the Rubins had founded the Juvenile Diabetes Foundation in order to raise money for Dr. Mintz's continued work which they felt might someday save their children. It was a sign.

We all agreed after carefully researching this researcher, that this was where the bequest should go. It turned out to be double the original sum. Thus began my relationship with Dr. Mintz, my parents' almost total involvement in the Foundation and a full decade in which there was to be for me a renewal of faith, an end to false hope and the family's submergence in the hectic, dedicated and ego-ridden world of charity.

In February of 1973, I came home from the Rice House in Durham, bitter and broken and not much caring to be mended. That period of mourning Dr. Norton had prescribed was a long one that degenerated into self-pity. With the encouragement of others, along with my own passion and endurance, I got out the Elmer's Glue-All and started to get myself together. I stopped examining the sick pieces and contemplated the whole shebang. With my newfound interest in fund-raising public appearances and my subsequent return and serious application to art, I faced reality and, of course, tried to improve on it. I found myself fashioning a positive public life out of the negatives of my private one.

I would now have a stage to be a ham on. And I would enjoy it. With experience came technique. You can even wear sackcloth with style. Slowly the image of the laughing, ever-noble, always positive, I-can-beat-anything Gary Kleiman emerged out of the ashes. And it's true, all of it. My life has been full and, in many ways, wonderfully satisfying. Even now, in this sorry state, I'm full of piss and vinegar. Anyone meeting me and not familiar with my story doesn't even think me sick, cannot even tell that I'm blind. And that's the way I want it. It's so weird and has always been.

One of my patients—I'll call him Erik—is a perfect example of diabetes's sneaky method. He's a blond bull of seventeen and a football player. He seems to have leaped out of one of those Nazi posters of a *Jungling*, an advertisement of Nordic superiority and power. His image could lure Adolf out of hell for another try at it. Erik is bursting with health—or so it seems. He evokes so many images. Surely the sweet bird of youth. And he's spilling sugar all over the place.

My patch of vision has become all-seeing, goddamnit, perhaps proving that the law of compensation is still on the books. I look at Erik and see myself a decade ago. I, too, had the world by the tail. I, too, was a jock. I find myself fusing with him, hoping to recycle my own life through him. Everything is selfish. It just depends on what makes you happy. I want to make his life better than mine. Erik is helping. He is a model patient. He does all the right things and maybe he can save us.

I trust, at least partially because of me, Erik's diet and testing pattern are well controlled. *His* trapeze act is in balance. With Erik, my function is simpler than with most kids. I encourage and commend his disciplines and I advise him on how better to balance his food and insulin intake before and after his strenuous games. He handles it all very well.

Despite his dedication, Erik worries about his future as well he can. I called from the hospital this morning for fear he had read an article about my operation and condition. He mustn't complicate his life with fear. Loss of hope can be as destructive as loss of control.

Erik! Seventeen! He's one of the lads who may, with luck, stave off the horrors for years. The wheel goes round and round and we've got to buck the percentages.

My own determination to beat the odds, to discover and realize any gifts I may possess, to live before I die became—as time went on—an obsession. I began to treasure and husband every second of the day, which I bemoaned only had twenty-four hours.

My fight for life became a crusade with standards flying.

One day, I don't know just when, the nonessentials fell away and I started living at my fullest potential. For better or worse, my life has become art. Tragic or comic, it's at least always dynamic, extreme, aiming high and in one direction. I haven't the time to aim anywhere else. I came to accept the fact that I could never be the boy next door. Diabetes has trained me for more glamorous environs—like left field or out on a limb or even to the borders of desperation but always in the limelight. It's a star turn.

Disease can be a drag that keeps one from moving gracefully through life or it can demand the concentration of energy that makes one soar. This isn't a romantic vision of disease but a practical use of it. When I sculpt, I chip away the unnecessary. I've done the same with what's left of my life. I want the ideal. With no time for the crap that clutters most of our stories. *Clean and simple.*

Characters in fine plays and novels say and do only the things that forward the plot and their development as heroes or villains. Hamlet had no time for hemorrhoids or Scarlett O'Hara torn underwear and hangnails. Neither of them in their frustrated quests wasted time on the garbage that litters most of our relationships. No Time for Shit should be the title of this book and my epitaph. If everyone would cut it out of their lives, what a world we'd have. But people play like

116

infants with shit, get lost in it and it colors their entire histories.

I have no *time* for shit and that has made me special and enviable. Nothing around me is superfluous and nothing I do is without purpose. If this sounds inhuman, perhaps it is. Spontaneity is not a probable adjunct of diabetes, although humor is certainly a necessary one. I am saved from being a health machine by my own wild spirit, lately captive and plotting and planning to be free again.

The race against death doesn't always bring out the best in a guy. Restlessness, impatience with anything less than perfect performance, fear or wariness of emotional commitment, physiological changes of mood do not make for tranquility. But who in hell wants tranquility? I seek challenge in relationships as well as everything else. Someone who won't take my crap, who makes like demands of mutual respect, depth of feeling, expansion of spirit. Without caring we're all doomed.

When I eventually got out of myself and took my place in the world, when I identified with others instead of demanding that they identify with me, it was a beginning.

I tell you, I've been lucky. My family has been the greatest, I its only discordant note. I was always a thing possessed, ticking away like a time bomb, eager to be released, seeking high adventure, more attention, not one dull moment. They are so damned perverse up there. Some of our dreams and prayers are too readily answered.

Yet my days have been full and productive. I can't wait until I get back to them full time. The days are wonderful, but when the guards are down at night and I lie in the dark, sometimes the terrible reality overcomes me, the enormity, the unbelievable audacity of the operation, the whole business, and it's then that I want to yell, "Where's the fucking manager?"

Just today, after being home again at my own place, I suddenly was inexplicably dehydrated, suffering for a change from hypotension which, right now, can be much more damaging than my *high* blood pressure. I was disgusted. They're so goddamned *endless,* the complications. So utterly relentless. A change in treatment will cure *this* and create still another problem. I feel like Job without his God.

Yes, it's at night when the anger sometimes changes to despair and awful thoughts take hold of me. In the dark of night I hug my doom to me like the lover I've rejected.

# 15

GROWING UP IN Miami Beach did not prepare one for the rigors of reality. If you lived anywhere near us, you had a house, a pool and a couple of cars. I mean, the oranges and grapefruits fell onto your breakfast table; you didn't even have to reach for them. The sun was shining, the palms were swaying, your Pa was rich and your Ma was good lookin'.

When I woke every morning, I could look across Indian Creek and my first sight was a storybook castle that glowed by day and glittered at night. It was like Oz for sure, a shimmering Hotel Fontainebleu. At the foot of my bed lay this extra dream, and like everything else, it was obtainable. By day, I could swim in its pool, play in its gardens and scoot around the lobby watching pale and rich northerners check in and bronze and relaxed ones check out. At night I could only dare to imagine the international espionage and romantic goings on in the moonlighted recesses of that sprawling pile of stone. Some day! I mean, some night! What a wonderful banquet was ahead of me.

I did know that, as a baby, we were so hard up that I ate canned spaghetti, but I didn't actually remember that, though Glenn and I were often reminded of it. I somehow had the idea that babies were born poor and as they aged they got richer and sicker—often simultaneously. It was a law of nature. Like graying and wrinkling. Using my own family's history, this was my belief.

If you lived long enough, you might hobble around complaining about your ailments but you were a millionaire and I supposed paid extravagantly for that long lease on life.

That was it. You started like Marty with a struggle that ended with victory and Vuitton luggage, a membership in a golf club, a beautifully dressed wife and fun sons who went to Ivy League colleges.

Any sights and sounds of poverty didn't register on our trips back and forth to Miami or wherever. If, after my father had found the pot of gold at the end of the rainbow, Marge had had a third son and if Lacoste had made diapers, the kid would have worn them—only once! We really were well cared for.

At sixteen—and less—all my pimply faced friends had a car and the parking lot at Miami Beach Senior High School, which was an eighteen-carat stone's throw from our house, looked like an auto show in the lobby of the Roney Plaza. I mean, practically everybody sat at the wheel of a Jaguar, Camaro, Porsche, Firebird, Mercedes Benz or a Caddy. Even more than the other kids, I was insulated. By the boundaries of my illness, my parents' resonating indulgence and, most of all, by my pre-Copernican conviction that the universe revolved around me. Because I was so exceptional, there was that little matter of my sickness—a nuisance but still unrevealed in all its ferocity. That sickness, according to my observation, was an anomaly, at my age. But I had always been different.

Even the very old died naturally in Miami Beach—in a condominium and sports clothes. They even came to Florida for that express purpose, only to find themselves on a milk train long past their station, banding together to create a majority block of voters with undying devotion to their city and the politicians who respected their needs. As long as they could make it to the polls, they were to be reckoned with. Everything was neat and in its place.

Yes. Until my complications, life was simple, egalitarian and available in every department. The world was a boutique where *reasonable* meant the least extravagant and *cheap* was a word no one would use. This was an ambience evidently funded by John MacArthur and Aristotle Onassis.

My parents decided that all of this was too rarefied for Glenn and me and I was transferred to Fisher Junior High, where I was introduced at last to peers who lived in the oh-too-real world. I saw up close my first blacks, my first slums and my first Plymouth. I also took a good look around when I heard, *"Mira! Mira!"* and saw plenty more. The scene was foreign with subtitles, but I catch on fast. I was hit over the head—and about time.

I was wheeled back into the transplant unit at Jackson Memorial Hospital yesterday because some bug drained me so that I couldn't move on my own. Bugs of all kind come to me now as if by prearrangement. So help me. I advertise. That's the nature of Cyclosporin. If I could barely call down to my mother to get my ass to the hospital, I, who refuse help reflexively, must have been half-dead. The "wing" and a prayer have me sitting up and taking notes again. A transfusion helped, too. Well, at least I don't have far to go when I return to work.

This hospital has been home, playground, workroom. But I wonder what I would be like without the Juvenile Diabetic Foundation, which I'd never heard of before Duke.

Those six Miami families with stricken children who had applied for and received a local charter of the JDF in 1971 now had, with that initial donation of ours, a new source of energy and imagination—my parents. In an effort to take diabetes out of the closet and alert the world to its dangers, this band of young, swinging marrieds decided that the National American Diabetes Association told people what they wanted to hear—that insulin could control the disease and we could all, as in *Never on Sunday*, happily go off to the seashore. Well, these Floridians didn't believe it. Each parent had a child who was still living proof. I, for one, had been on insulin religiously for thirteen years and was then and now in a state of decay. No. The answer was not insulin, but a cure. A cure meant research and research meant money.

As the JDF thought the ADA was too complacent, there is no

doubt they thought us too sensational. Bob Kronowitt, an original live wire whose daughter Tracy was also diabetic, was so creative and so responsive to Dr. Mintz's needs that he was encouraged to go professional and be paid to work exclusively for the Foundation. He was convinced that the public had to be shocked by making the terrible intelligence available. He felt, and we all agreed, that justifiable fear instead of false hopes would raise the necessary loot. It was a matter not only of approach but of intent. The American Diabetes Association believed in protecting the family and not being alarmist. I'm not so sure that it isn't because of us—as well as finer tuning—that they now have removed the sugar coating and also admit diabetes is a killer.

All I know is that our initial donation, and the reflexive invitation to my parents to join the board, changed our lives and rocked the Foundation. My mother didn't believe it when she heard about Casino Night, where the Foundation transformed the Jockey Club into Monte Carlo with twenty-five dollars' worth of Monopoly money. Marge is nothing if not big time, and those penny-ante days were soon to be in the past. Pennies were not going to save lives fast enough. Not that Marge and Marty hadn't joined forces with some pretty dynamic people. I just think that, as the hottest new additions, they really made the pot steam and whistle even more.

Nothing is simple in this world except some people, and the simplest of them is complex as hell. All these couples were activated by their frustration and their need to alter the inevitable. They cared about all children. Secretly, of course, each couple prayed that some discovery, some serum, some miracle that would reverse the irreversible would save their own son or daughter. If not, others might eventually be helped. Damnit, I think these people are great.

I say this knowing that—as with all do-gooders—there are less admirable drives that corrupt and cause collision. How do you get creative, energetic, substantial people in one room with one common goal and not at the same time collect a bouquet of clashing egos and bruisable psyches that can smell to high heaven? It's the whole cherry without the pit business. It can't be done and one has only to wonder at the good done by such admixtures and not belabor the temperament that sired it. The saints themselves were not free of self-congratulation as they languished in terminal virtue and the national JDF or our present JDRF (Juvenile Diabetes Research Foundation), no more than the UN, the AMA, the YMCA and the ASPCA are not saints but men and women who are *trying*.

I'm a great believer in doing, and with all the fuming and sparking, these vibrant young couples along with my parents managed to aim high and in the right direction. It might have been that diabetes was the new cause and therefore something to hitch a social wagon to. It might have been, as the membership blessedly became larger, some bored and rich lady's escape from the drudgery of shopping Worth Avenue. It might have been an otherwise repressed talent's chance to display. It might have been any of these things and worse, but damnit, so what? They are evolved human beings concentrating their energy, acting in concert and for the common good, and I, a grateful recipient, say thank you for being frail and funny and human and helping us.

Some of these colorful people live in fantasy worlds and make them come true—quite a feat outside of padded cells. Some are truly off-the-wall crazy and thank God aren't in those cells, because we need their bursting vitality.

In this world of cellars and playrooms and folding chairs and ice water, excited, motivated young glamour girls motivated other parents to insure the future of countless children, some still unborn. Countless numbers that touchingly always have come down to the specific one each is really talking about.

Astonishingly, all workers became parent to the child and all children belonged to the one member. That little group was radiant, its rays reaching out to the JDF groups in Philadelphia and in Washington, D.C., and New Jersey. These self-made men and their stylish wives would seem to have been the least likely recruits for a crusade. But underneath the suntans, jewelry and

Gucci finery were the pale and nagging ghosts of their once-healthy children. Was the disease that hit their young a punishment for their own hard-earned indulgences? Had they offended the Boss? And, if so, couldn't they reverse the orders by taking over the business themselves? Like my father, most of these men worked for themselves and got things done if no one else would do it. Vital, aggressive and fanatical amateurs, these couples started with raffles and wine-tasting parties and were thrilled to get a hundred dollars from an airline pilot whose son was another statistic.

Ninety percent of this and everything else went to research. Costs were somehow unbelievably defrayed so that even after the Foundation became big business, it still distributed at least eighty percent of its gross donations. A miracle if you examine other organizations from the Red Cross down. The percentages are almost—if not—reversed. This has always been a dedicated group, the JDRF. From raising eighteen hundred dollars in one year, back in 1972, they now realize seven figures, but like diabetes it took its toll on the family. The Foundation was to become so time-consuming that it started taking over our lives in an effort to save mine.

When my parents get involved, there's no cutting corners, ever. The JDF, once my parents were on board, was destined to take off. *Eighteen hundred dollars?* my parents thought testily. Their initial contribution of ten thousand dollars was soon supplemented by the tremendous public response to the Chusmir article in the *Herald*. When it attracted another twelve thousand in one week, Bob Kronowitt knew that he had in me the making of a star.

The federal government, after rescinding the fifty thousand dollars earmarked for Dr. Mintz and his beta cell research, had left the good doctor with that eighteen hundred dollars, and Bob Kronowitt, who could draw rabbit stew out of a hat, asked what else he could use. With a sad smile, Dr. Mintz had helplessly replied, "Ten thousand, at least." It was his, and then the next twelve as well.

124

Things started to happen rapidly. On schedule, as if it had all been written. The ten-thousand dollar bequest from the estate did turn out to be nearer to twenty-five, and now my parents, accepting the JDF"s invitation, were firmly on the board. And they didn't just sit there. My parents don't know how to sit. In no time flat, Marge became fund-raising chairwoman and my father, executive vice-president. And they produced: from that day when Nancy Marumsrud Kahn (who only recently died in that terrible Louisiana plane crash) motioned and got seconded a twenty-five-dollar petty-cash fund to later days when Robert Held, Sr., guaranteed a quarter of a million dollars for a diabetic chair (so self-effacingly in his daughter-in-law Mary Lou's name) and the remarkable Polly de Hirsch Meyer, still very much with us, left us one million dollars in trust payable on her death but borrowable in a crisis.

These dynamos were working overtime. From what Marge considered PTA meetings to a nationally recognized competitive force in medical philanthropy, there have been ten years of back-breaking work. The original dream of a research center became a real institute where I work; and our patron saint, Dr. Daniel H. Mintz, has now been honored with a million-dollar chair—the first in diabetic inquiry. A trip like that has to start with a first step, and that first step had better be in the right direction.

# 16

LIFE IS SO CRAZY. I mean, really bizarre. On the board with my parents—preceding them—was a woman who did *not* have a diabetic child. This was not the only thing about her that was unique. Ilene Luby was more a natural phenomenon than anything else, a storm that galvanized the whole community to action and reaction. Her very nice husband, Sam, was the Chevrolet distributor for Washington, Baltimore and Miami, and they had many friends and connections. Ilene's life was as eccentric as a Fellini movie and she was always appropriately costumed, jeweled and made up, always ready for her close-up. She and my mother always looked like movie stars to me, only Ilene would play a countess or something. She seems to live permanently in a scenario which she writes herself, and she makes every goddamn thing come true. She's really something. According to Marge, without Ilene Luby it would have taken an extra ten years to accomplish what was done. The woman works in broad strokes.

In 1973 she invited to lunch, along with fellow board members, ten of the most influential women in Dade County. Having lassoed them, she revealed her plan for an underwritten luncheon, with every member contributing to the seed-money affair. They all found themselves participating—one couple donating the flower arrangements, another the ballroom space, another the food and so on. The rookie Kleimans did the very stylish invitations.

This affair was to be held at the Coconut Grove Hotel and each couple charged one hundred or, as donors, two hundred dollars. The JDF was to realize a lot of dough—all of it because of an inspiration of Ilene's and, of course, impossible without the wild generosity of everyone else involved. Its success was to anticipate the annual Love and Hope Ball, a brilliant charity affair that has succeeded in rousing tremendous interest in diabetes and also the capital to fight it. The Board of Directors had now thrust the Foundation into public consciousness.

I demean no one when I report that since diabetes had indeed become the "in" disease I was, therefore the most stylish of young men. And so I was asked to speak at that first luncheon at the Grove. What better way to raise bread than to have a blind teenager illustrating the need?

Since Marge and Marty were so enthusiastic and the proceeds were for Dr. Mintz, I readily agreed. His work on beta cells, so demonstrable on rats, was to prove—because of the more complex immunization system of human beings—ineffective, but at that time there was hope. There is still hope as more sophisticated methods abound. The University of Miami's Diabetes Research Institute is presently second to none.

As I've made clear, there's nothing I wouldn't do for this man. In fear and depression, I would call him constantly and his kindness and patience never faltered. This is unchanged after ten years. "Just hang in there, Gary," he has always said and here I am—my neck a little longer, my body still short. Somehow though, my noose became a lifeline.

I was eager to help the cause, but a night before the luncheon it happened. The whole gang was in our kitchen. My parents, Glenn and Robin and I. We were making ersatz, saltless pizza with tomatoes and peppers and there was flour all over the place. We were turning out colored glue instead of pasta. Everybody was laughing and having a ball and I was dancing around like a maniac when all of a sudden I saw it. It was the tiniest black dot, like a pinpoint hole in the eye.

"Oh, my God! No," I screamed as the dot became a spot became a lake and then a river. It spread quickly, and as I went into panic, Robin held me just whispering, "No, no. It mustn't." The rest of the gang scattered to call the doctor, the hospital, prepare my bed. I felt the panic in everyone—and the pity in Robin's voice. The bleeding was bad enough without that.

"Please go home, Robin. Don't make a big thing of this. Everybody leave me alone, *please*. I've got to lie down."

Then I made my way to bed, sitting up, being very still and waiting for it to subside. Instead it got worse. I watched what looked like a drop of ink in water, only thicker—about the consistency of jellyfish—spreading across the entire eye. If I shook it, there was a kind of delayed motion.

When it happens, it's hard not to worry it, test it, almost play with it. It's almost as if you're controlling it, but you're not. It's like stopping a flood by putting a bamboo screen in its path. Nothing. But it's fascinating. If you move too quickly or shake your head, the blood spurts anew like a slow-motion stream, and everywhere it travels it obliterates, displacing sight.

I had learned that with everything there is a range of good to bad, and I remember the intensity of my pleas. *Make it a good, a little hemorrhage. Please don't make it a big bad one.* My heart sank as it got worse, but I kept hoping the damage wouldn't be total. There was nothing else for me to do but hope and pray at this point. No specialist could have done more than my family. It's one of the many moments when you are alone. *Please don't make it a big one. Don't make the damage total.* Anything less was good news and welcome.

It's one way of going to sleep, praying. When I awoke in the morning, my well-trained body was still in exactly the same position I had carefully assumed at night. After so many hours, the blood usually settles. This time it had not. To wake up and not wake up filled me with horror. I heard my father's voice, felt the mattress yield to the pressure of his weight. I opened my eyes wide and was totally blind.

128

"It's all over, Dad."

I really thought it was good-bye, Charlie, and then I heard my mother at the door. When my father repeated what I'd said, she came rushing in. I really thought, we all thought, it was the end. Glenn was suddenly on the bed leaning over me, kissing me. The whole family was sobbing and stroking me, and I thought, I will never let this happen again. My family must never go through this one more time. If I'm blind I'm blind, and *if* the eye comes back, I will suffer the next blackout by myself. I'll ride it out alone—at least with no additional dialogue.

What was left of my sight in my left eye returned slowly, but obviously I was unable to make the luncheon. Though the bleeding had stopped, I had to lie very still.

Through Ilene's influence, a few celebrities were to appear, but I was to have been the terrible centerpiece of the banquet, the specter at the feast, the "shill" to attract the moola. And there I was in hospital, as Monty Python would say. Ilene was undaunted. If I couldn't attract contributions by drawing tears that would moisten the ferns and salt the almonds, she came up with a better idea. She never stops.

"Why don't you speak, Marge?"

"What?"

"I mean it, darling. It's a wonderful idea."

"Have you lost your mind completely?"

"Actually, the more I think about it, the more I believe the Fates have stepped in."

"They can step right out," Marge objected.

"But don't you see that under the circumstances—"

"That's it. I can't think of anything but Gary . . . you don't know."

"Convey it," Ilene urged.

"Of course, I'll convey it. That's all I'm thinking about."

"They'll eat it with a spoon."

"Ilene."

"Marge. You're his mother, and who else knows the needs of these kids better, can convince them more? I tell you it's an inspiration."

"My God. How can I?"

"Easily. You'll just be your natural self."

"Natural in front of that mob. I'll be so nervous."

"The more nervous you are the more natural. That's good."

"Oh, Ilene, for God's sake. I'm supposed to go on between Eva Marie Saint and Ted Shawn?"

"Are we going to have billing trouble now?" Ilene concluded.

"What can I say, Marty? How can I—" she said later in panic.

"You'll be great. Remember there'll be about two hundred people," Marty teased.

"Thanks a heap. Two hundred people!"

"Make believe you're picking up a Tony, honey."

"Thanks, this is not *Two for the Seesaw* or *Voice of the Turtle* for Uta Hagan's class. It's for Gary and the Coconut Grove Hotel and it's—"

Marty smiled gently. "Marge, babe. Just speak from your heart and it'll be fine."

And, oh, she did and it was. Ilene was right. They did eat it with a spoon. While I lay in bed, Mom realized why she was replacing me, why I had initially been asked in the first place; and even Dr. Mintz freaked out. He told me there wasn't a dry eye in the joint. Even he got out the handkerchief. "Broadway's loss," I've always said, having listened to subsequent appearances.

This was the first of many talks my mother gave, and that luncheon netted the JDF over forty thousand dollars. The food was great, the loot pure gravy for my scientific but emotional pal, Daniel Mintz and his Institute.

Accepted on the board of JDF in January 1973, Marge and Marty Kleiman by February were really up to their ears. Examining the minutes of those meetings it's a wonder that Marty's business and Marge's home survived their preoccupation. I tell you Glenn and I were sick of the whole business. They ate, drank and, at night, dreamed Foundation. I guess I forgot why they were there and almost resented their abstract devotion to me. God protect the family of anyone with a Cause no matter what—even if it's you. And if *I* felt this way one can only shudder at my brother's reaction.

From that first nervous making appearance, Marge became Miami's favorite heartbreaker. Luncheons and then, eventually, the annual Love and Hope Ball at two hundred and fifty a couple helped—of course only with the warm responsive Miami Beach crowd—to raise a fortune.

None of this was done without sacrifice. Though I was the initial reason for the involvement, I had no idea that my mother—whose main object in life up to now was to bug me— was now to have a surrogate career. I mean, things were changing. Like Bob and Micki Kronowitt with their little daughter, they and the rest of the other parents were on fire. Informed by federal statistics that juvenile diabetes allowed at most a life span of only twenty-seven years after onset, they had to move fast. The miracle of Jonas Salk's serum was not lost on these mothers and fathers. Imagine being crippled from infantile paralysis the day the cure was made public? It would be like dying on Armistice Day. Everyone was gratified by the newly appointed laboratory at the hospital and its subsequent unit. Everyone was amazed that my hometown's realistic annual goal was soon to become three hundred thousand dollars compared with the national five million. Everyone was proud that Miami was now really on the map. Philadelphia wanted us to join them and become part of a national JDF. In no time at all. These few people were really achievers.

Glenn and I made our parents sign a contract that they would drop all talk of the Foundation and refuse all phone calls at mealtimes. The medium had really taken over the message and we were reeling from their twenty-four-hour-a-day commitments.

I was in and out of hospitals and under constant medication and, when well enough, making appearances for the Foundation. Glenn was being his own mother and father as well as brother to the prince for whom all this feverish activity was designed. He didn't have anything dramatic enough to cure, unless we all devoted ourselves to a war against patient acquiescence and martyrdom.

Except for several months as young boys, when we shared one bedroom for the first and last time, my brother and I were always close. We'd always gotten on so well that our parents had no reason to believe we wouldn't have a ball living in the same room. That specific familiarity, however, although it might not have bred contempt, did bring about a bloody civil war. I guess, all things considered, Glenn had needed his very own space to lick his wounds and compose himself. And now he'd been robbed even of that. It was soon over—that period—and we were again the Corsican brothers. Our eyebrows would raise simultaneously when the phone would ring and our loving household was again invaded.

This was the time of the great and reversed decision. There was that great pressure for the JDF—as it was still called—to go national, for us in Miami and Philadelphia, Washington, D.C., and southern New Jersey to join forces, which we eventually did. It was tempting for obvious reasons, all financial. The clout, the prestige would be tremendous. We were effective, we were wanted. For those six or seven original families, this was the big time, like Hawaii and Alaska becoming part of the United States of America. What was resistible was our loss of control in funding. It would be catch as catch can for Dr. Mintz and his dedicated search for a cure.

The national JDF promised to refund all monies we raised in the first year, but after that we would have to feed the mother organization; an advisory board would specify which programs were viable and Philadelphia was apparently to have been the powerful, decisive force.

There was some disagreement as to which would be more deserving since "federal" and "state," as it were, had different thrusts. It *was* really like states' rights, I guess. We in Miami wanted the best of two possible worlds, but most important was the immediacy of a cure through research. As seen in my dramatic physical complications, the JDF was offered proof positive that, life-saving though insulin was, its religious use did not necessarily preclude the satanic violation of the patient's body. We

132

were considered alarmist in our attempt to make diabetes less innocuous and reveal it as the "Quiet Killer." We addressed ourselves first to the *quality* of life and its all too well-observed diminution.

In precise terms, the other couples saw me at nineteen and refused to believe that *their* children would end up the same way. Some of the kids were three and six and eight. Ten or fifteen years of dedicated research could conceivably save them. But it had to be fast. And so there was this immediacy in Miami. Marge and Marty Kleiman, already clobbered, still wanted me around ten years hence in case the miracle occurred.

If only we could have remained national and kept our sovereignty, but, alas, it ain't the way things go. We thought we could, but we couldn't. We were part of the mainstream for about five minutes, because at that time the ADA believed that the admittedly life-saving serum discovered by Drs. Banting and Best made an immediate cure unnecessary, that psychological acceptance of diabetes and proper control of it through instruction had first priority. Our local chapter couldn't buy this.

It took years for the ADA to say that we generated a revolution that declared loud and clear that diabetes was a killer and not a "controllable disease." Since those days, their practical concern for education and control has been just great.

At that time, Banting and Best, using the pancreases of sheep, simulated the insulin the sick human organ ceases to make sufficiently—if at all—in order to promote the utilization of food in the body. Without their extraordinary gift to humankind, I would not be here greedily wanting more for myself and the kids I work with. There's so little time once the subtle changes take place.

Dr. Best himself was one of those who accused us of being sensationalists. Dr. George Heffner, a leading pediatrician and diabetologist, said darkly that we were stirring people up.

Bob Kronowitt, aware of my hemorrhaging, always fearing for his daughter, answered him formally.

"Your patients, Doctor, are being attacked organ by organ. We would rather scare the patient into the strictest discipline and the powers into financing the quickest possible cure than face the inevitability of joyless youth and premature death."

When a national meeting took place in Philadelphia and my parents attended, a board member rose in answer to these arguments.

"Well, it's true, we may not be able to cure our children, but certainly we will our *grand*children!"

That did it. The schism was soon complete. The word *children* had no reality. If the JDF became richer for my parents' involvement, it was not only in fund raising. More importantly, Marge and Marty made human a humane organization. They gave a name and a force to abstract numbers. The scourge was recognizable in me. And it may be that emotional parents instead of scientists were meant to make board decisions. At any rate, for better or worse, that was the personality of our local Foundation. Not professionals but wild, caring families with a common bond and goal. It wasn't a cartel but—big as it became—it remained a family business. It's really neat.

I can hear Marge now. "If it takes robbing a bank or tying ourselves to the White House fence, we'll get the money and we'll get the cure." And the rest of that great gang is all of the same mind. There were those who believed that for all our independence it might be a mistake to secede. I remember someone saying that in our chauvinism and in our parochialism we had settled for being Dolphins fans. But it all worked out just fine. Any football fan will corroborate my news that settling for our Dolphins is no mistake.

While we were momentarily national, and didn't have the word *research* in our title, Congress was soliciting information from interested parties while a committee was considering an appropriation for diabetic research. I was asked by our group to speak—actually to be Exhibit A. I guess if I couldn't get a buck out of the committee, no one could. I pulled myself out of my torpor and let Bob Kronowitt and my father take me to Washington.

I packed my drug store, some rice, some wild cherry Life Savers and my sullen psyche and we were off to the capital. I know I must have been more impressed than I was admitting. After all, Washington was the seat of our government and a beautiful town, even with—or perhaps because of—my fractional vision, a classical metropolis, kind of jazzed up and peopled by the common folk in slacks and sweaters.

You looked at the pure white buildings and large spaces and you kind of visualized high-minded senators in white togas and laurel wreaths. That is, you saw that if you were a romantic idiot. From the facts, Congress was a House of a different color; still, I was somewhat in awe as I waited in what looked like a small wood-paneled courtroom with a long desk where the committee sat with, as I recall, Old Glory behind them. Bob or my father whispered, "They wouldn't give a damned penny for cancer some years ago and half the committee is dead of it." Typical.

I listened to the proceedings almost numbed by their dullness. I had imagined a dramatic scene of passionate requests that inspired loud refusals or heartfelt grants, breathtaking in their generosity. All of this directed with pacing and dispatch. All of it in high style. Brother! They were all so boring. The endless statistics, the packaged solicitude. The formality.

"Oh, thank you, Mr. Kronowitt. You have been most helpful. How can we convey our gratitude, sir—"

"Mr. Kleiman, we will not lose the faith, sir. We want you to know how pleased we are that you have diabetes—if we could only communicate our sympathy and pleasure in seeing you in Washington in such a terrible condition, sir."

"One can only hope, sir, that with our great interest—"

No one has ever heard so many sir's except perhaps at the bestowal of honors on Queen Elizabeth's birthday.

I remember names like Carter and Symington, Rogers, Vander Jagt and Heinz. All of them oppressively pleasant.

Bob's statement was compact and impressive. One billion dollars in health funds appropriated by Congress had not been spent by the health-related agencies of the Department of

Health, Education and Welfare. To Bob and the rest of the board—if not the present committee—it seemed unreasonable that the money be lying fallow while over ten million juvenile diabetics could be saved from not-so-slow deterioration.

Politesse and protocol gave way to blood and guts when Bob spoke. Before that it was hard to take sides, everything was so boring. When my name was called, I came alive. I felt my father touch me gently and I rose to walk the short distance to the desk appointed the witness. I had studied the layout of the place, as I do all new restaurants and strange places. Once I was set on my path, I thought, *They want statistics, I'll give them one.*

I walked bravely, my head erect, and stumbled just before I reached my goal. I heard a collective gasp and hoped only that my father wouldn't interpret it as a reaction or something negative. I knew I was being outrageous, but I couldn't repress the urge. Anyway, I had to do it and hoped Marty would understand. He did. He had sired a ham.

My quick recovery and valiant refusal to be helped brought a little tragic relief to the whole comedy. I think they were all grateful to be able to cut through all the bullshit and feel a little something. You know I looked so healthy that I had to gild the lily that was so prematurely placed in my hands.

My father copied down what I said that day. The fooling around was over.

> Gentlemen. You'll have to excuse my not having a prepared statement, but if I had one, I couldn't read it. I am going blind from diabetes. When I was six years old I became one of the statistics you've been hearing about. A child with diabetes. Then at eighteen I was another statistic, a young man with complications from diabetes. I now can become another statistic. There is no choice. I can be one of the stricken who will be dead ten years from now or I can be the best statistic of all—a person cured of diabetes. By funding the necessary research, you can make *that* possible.

It still sounds pretty good to me, but all the soft soap couldn't clean out the U.S. Treasury. What we eventually got was an appropriation of an appropriation instead of an outright allocation. Cancer and diabetes don't quite have the attractive immediacy of weaponry.

The flourishing, little Foundation was on its own. God helps those, etcetera, etcetera. I couldn't feel too guilty about my performance.

Nancy Marumsrud had us advertised all over Miami on a Goodyear blimp and she asked me to do spot commercials for the Foundation. I was reluctant at first, it seemed so tacky; but I knew the importance of such publicity.

It came easily and I quickly accepted the necessary showmanship that helps persuade. I guess I was always a realist. When I was little, I used to make five wishes for myself before sleep. Then as a backup, I would make five wishes for everybody else in the world so I wouldn't be considered selfish and consequently get nothing. I started conning the guys upstairs very early on.

Anyway, after the second session, I not only warmed to the telecasts but became a pro. Appearing on TV, I found, wasn't too bad at all, except that the ordinarily earthy crew was so fucking solicitous that I thought I'd freak out. I was being treated with all the awe and respect usually reserved for the freshly dead.

People treat serious illness—in others, of course—as if it were some kind of accomplishment that humbles the unafflicted. It's so dumb. It's so boring. And so when they were taking my voice levels and I had to rehearse my lines for the millionth time, I rewrote them.

"My name is Gary Kleiman and I'm here to say that diabetes is the foremost cause of homosexuality and traffic jams in this great country of ours."

There was a hoot and a yell and that was the end of all the reverential crap.

The minute spots we did for the Foundation, more reasonably composed, were intended to enlighten the public and invite contributions, and, since it was important that I do them, I enjoyed myself. Not my father, who made several with me. In the first place, he was ill at ease in front of a camera. And then he almost choked on the words he was asked to say in reference to the federal cutoff of funds, "Cure diabetes before it kills my son—or yours." And more difficult still, "It will not only be a personal loss but a national disgrace if my son dies."

As a matter of fact, I could have killed *him*. He couldn't get the words out and there must have been a million takes. My toughness comes from my mother. Poor Marty would be doing just fine, and then would come the heavy stuff, "My son is going to—"

I always thought that if they had kept shooting and printed one of those takes in which he broke up, we might have raked in a fortune.

This was a job and I removed myself from the reality. Marty couldn't. He kept me in the blasted warehouse all day. That was where Channel 4 had its studio. In my attempt to give the crew what it wanted, I ignored the text and concentrated on the mechanics. I could always horse around, but what was this fucking career—exploiting my misery for whatever lofty reason? That couldn't be the entire point of my existence. Anyway, there was also something tainted about my self-advertisement. I got too much satisfaction—grisly though it might have been—from hamming it up. It was a real bad time, 1973. I was a hell of a mess—laughing or crying.

My mother and father, through their rapidly accelerating involvement with the Juvenile Diabetes Research Foundation, were managing to some extent to exorcise the demons that had invaded our home. No matter how indirect or abstract, they were doing something for me and others like me. They were moving, activated. I was just wallowing and displaying myself like a freak.

When you're in there fighting, details blessedly take over. There is no time for agonizing in the midst of battle. The business of defense and attack replaces the reasons. Sitting at home waiting for the news is the bitch. Negotiating with your neighbors, bargaining for ammunition and setting up the task of building a fort along with others who have a common fear but disparate needs and clashing personalities engage your energies to such a degree that purpose is lost in the doing. I wasn't ready.

I meant what I said about being lucky—about my living at my greatest potential. Who knows what tomorrow will bring? But sometimes, like right this minute, when my creatinine has gone up without apparent reason and I'm back in the hospital for a look-see, I dream of going back somehow to that fatal moment to undo whatever it was that gave me diabetes, that keeps me on a twenty-four-hour alert. It's not a very practical or satisfying fantasy. I'm always fighting the undertow and—once in a while—I'm tempted to surrender to it.

The thing is, I can't. My arms and legs thrash about; I stay afloat and I emerge a hero again. But it's not bravery. It's simply reflex. I was born to fight. My history is made up of nothing but Agincourts, Yorktowns and Bunker Hills. A string of stunning victories that deny the reality of preparations, sieges and retreats. I've been at war all my life and my resources are still undrained.

In short, the toll on others as I fight my war is heavy. The list of casualties breaks my heart while I keep charging, my loyal and loving army close behind. There are times, however, like this minute, when the damned shining armor seems to have adhered to my skin and I and twelve surgeons can't remove it. I'd like some rest. I'd like an air bath. I'm sick of war and nobility. And between you and me, I'm scared. To hell with flaming, gleaming swords. There are split seconds when I simply want to smash my fists against the hospital wall and then cry because they hurt and it didn't do any good and I can then admit to being helpless.

I want desperately to be that human, but I can't. No way. If I want to survive, I mustn't allow more than a pinch of self-pity. It will pass, this rage, because I've written it down and given it shape—a shape that can be discarded once seen. Yes, the fury will abate and I'll laugh again. I'll die laughing. Yes, I'll go home and be funny and sunny and try to light up the dark. But I don't want to be like the sun. The sun is uninhabitable. I want to be a warm and hospitable place. Jesus, I'm marinated in love and, because of that, designed to give pain to everybody close to me. And so that red light that I switch on when I traffic with the ladies.

If I see this fucking hospital room once more, they'll have to tie me up. I want to get up to New York or San Francisco or maybe Vermont, where Marge is fixing up a summer place for us all. Summer! It seems so distant, perhaps unattainable. Even the seasons are goals now. I remember thinking, *Will I see Carter or Reagan as President? Will I see America beat the Russians in the Olympics? Will I see the hostages safely home from Iran? Will I see the Skylers' expected baby?* And now, will I see morning?

The only things in life I have found predictable are diabetes and my mother. They have never fallen short of my expectations. I can depend on them with certainty, and even death and taxes cannot compare with their immutability. If you're shrewd and fast, you can evade both of them for a time. Except for diabetes mellitus and Marge Kleiman, I am happy to report that there are flaming loopholes everywhere and my circus act extends to jumping through them unscathed.

# 17

IT'S NO SECRET that people can be shitty and self-interested, as well as noble and self-interested, but, damnit, you can't pigeonhole them as I once thought. I mean, just as you think you've met a prize-winning bastard, he comes through in the most breathtaking reversal of character. A devoted slave whose unquestioning loyalty is almost contemptible changes his name to Spartacus. It's just great.

To someone who sculpts, who sets a form in space for whatever "forever" is, it's notable that only in art is anything permanently fixed. Others have come before me, like Calder, whose notion it was to imitate life with sculpture that is always on the move, kinetically subject to the currents around it. Still, for me, the vision, the attainable goal and its subsequent performance, is what art is about. I mean, imagine a balding David or a Praxiteles athlete gone to pot. Imagine a frowning Mona Lisa recalling some former slight. I happily doubt that Adam and God will make the Sistine Chapel a scene of Indian wrestling, although secularly it has come to that. No. Art is long and steady. It is life that is all surprise. Just as you've got a situation down pat, whammo! It keeps you on your toes.

When I returned from Duke, it was one bloody mess after another. I was hemorrhaging pretty regularly, having laser-beam treatments and very negative prognoses. I was filled with fear, bitterness and a kind of black phony stardom. Having seen the annual cerebral palsy marathon shows on TV, I now felt like their crippled child with a new lyric to the song. *Look at me, I'm stumbling.* My future had obviously slipped through my fingers. Nipped in the bud, my life was on hold. I hadn't grown into the part yet or found my costume.

When I knew that a return to Syracuse was out of the question, I slept a lot and listened to stacks of sentimental, easy, identifiable rock. Bob Dylan was fabulous, but too cynical for me. James Taylor, Joni Mitchell, Dan Fogelberg and, especially, Jackson Browne kept me wallowing. I strummed my guitar, idly vamping until the finale. I was a zombie, filling my life with other things because love and life seemed beyond my grasp.

I saw little. There was less in the future. I gave myself my tests and shots by rote, bitched a lot and dumbly watched TV like Dylan, my pup. In the most horrible kind of galactic way, I was drifting like a hapless astronaut into space, away from the mother ship, away from all life.

Then out of the cobalt blue I heard that Gene Massin had asked where I had disappeared to and, if I were around, for me to drop in and see him. It was my only offer and I took him up on it. Gene really reached unreachable me. He became my first mentor.

A massive man with massive sons of his own and an outsize appetite for life as well as work, Gene had a lot of iron-gray hair and shrewd, black eyes. They seemed to see everything hidden from sight. He loved an audience and I was a one-man claque. He talked and I listened, and what I heard made me return every day between our classes. I just showed up at his studio, which was a combination smithy, home, museum and social hall. I barely remember his nice wife, Helen, who seems to have gotten run over in all the traffic.

For about three months, I would look forward to seeing Gene daily and being part, no matter how peripherally, of this busy art world. It was the high point of my terrible day. Gene was too big a guy to pussyfoot around, so we talked about blindness.

"What does it look like, Gar?"

"Nothing."

"What does 'nothing' look like?"

"Like mud, I guess, nothing."

"What does mud look like?"

"I guess—well, it has different colors—murky colors."

"Then you don't see nothing, you see mud!"

"Big deal. What a view!"

But I started to elaborate.

"As a matter of fact, Gene, I've got a real gloomy extravaganza going when I hemorrhage. My own private Rorschach. Lots of inky blues and even streaks of silver."

"Shapes as well as colors, aren't they?"

"I guess so."

"So don't give me this 'nothing' shit."

Gene had a way with words—and with young people. He was just great with me. My own Dade County guru. We discussed what I laughingly called my future and he just hurdled my realism and spoke of my possibly going into sculpture, since my other current interest, psychology—like my other dreams of veterinary medicine and architecture—demanded my being what Glenn, not I, was. A bookworm.

"Sculpture," I shouted. "I don't even know what it is. I mean, I know *The Thinker* and Greek athletes and Venus without her arms but, come on."

Gene took me outside to his yard and showed me a small Styrofoam piece his son had cast in aluminum. He had been worrying it into several rough and polished surfaces.

"This is design, shape and texture. You can *feel* all of them. I think you'd be at home with form."

I felt the surfaces and he turned on a belt sander so I could feel the changes and follow the refinements. I still had sufficient vision between hemorrhages to get the whole picture. But sighted or not, I loved the idea of texture. And sculpture seemed to have better hours than psychology.

"I've been thinking, Gary. I'd like to introduce you to somebody. She hasn't been over lately, she's been so busy. But tomorrow—well, keep it open."

And that was my second step.

I met Audrey Corwin Wright, the oldest hippy I ever came across. Fabulous. A very good sculptor who worked in a variety of media. She was painting her refrigerator that afternoon when Gene and I made our way through the kitchen of her sprawling, art-filled studio house in Coconut Grove. Her structures large and small crowded each other out of the house into her garden, making a path like the giant banyan tree which was slowly marching across the property—as banyans have a habit of doing. The crazy ramshackled look of the place, the junglelike foliage, the makeshift furniture, the outdoor kiln and lifetime collection of mementos and drawings and comestibles that met my fractional gaze indoors and out will remain with me always.

"This is Gary Kleiman, Audrey."

And she kept working away on her refrigerator as if it were designed to keep the Last Supper fresh. I saw the whites of her eyes when she finally turned and looked up.

"Here's the deal," this Yankee lady announced. "There are eight-week sessions. If you don't like me, you leave. If I don't like you, you leave. If we outgrow each other, you leave."

*My God,* I thought. *I just got here, I don't want to go anywhere.*

I started the next day. It was the first of many. I would bring my insulin, Kempner's puffed rice and fruit each morning at nine and I would stay until five. Audrey saw my need and let me stay all day. My mother would drop me off and collect me like the family laundry, but I wasn't just hanging around, haunting the doctors or sleeping. I loved it at Audrey's.

At the end of that first day, she gave me a couple of chips of delicate, translucent alabaster. "Here! Do something with these." And she gave me some little tools. It was unbelievable, the feeling I got when a kind of abstract poodle emerged from the stone. I half-expected to hear an abstract bark. I loved what happened, and proudly brought my work to her the next day. Audrey was amazed and examined the piece carefully, turning it upside down and nodding her approval. "Not bad—not bad at all—interesting shape; but it's better this way, isn't it?" And it was. It now looked more—well—human and was far more felicitous in form.

144

Audrey taught me not to be satisfied, to be selective, to develop my taste. Most importantly, she taught me that there was more than one way to look at something. It had taken a while.

I loved using my hands, transforming objects, altering space. And I reveled in the sheer physicality of sculpting. That first caress of the virgin stone and then the remarkable sensation when my fingers felt the first signs of life. I ran out of chips and my father took me down to the ocean's edge so I could find pretty stones I could transform. I brought them like shiny apples to my teacher, only to learn they were not carvable. I loved seeking and sometimes finding approval from this teacher. And, more than anything, I loved working.

Every single day, along with a group of what I then thought of as old women, I worked in Audrey's garden. I was the elderly man and we worked away modeling, filing and hammering like hobgoblins in a fairy tale. Audrey, like Gene, was a worker and I caught the habit. For the first time in my life, my days were structured creatively rather than just cluttered pharmaceutically; and instead of bemoaning my seventy-five percent loss of vision, I was productively using what was left.

Audrey was something else. In teaching me both the rudiments and refinements of sculpture, she would say, "The best way to discern a shape, Gary, is to close one eye and squint with the other." Unbelievable! "You mean like this, Audrey?" I would say, opening my eyes as wide as possible. But it was great that she forgot—or didn't care.

I found another home away from home at Audrey's. There was always work and a lot of action, and I was part of still another family with my instructor and her charming British husband, Tom, who was a quickly relating, warm, undriven man who seemed in harmony with all things natural. He and his little plot of land were beautifully cultivated. His flowers were beautiful. These apparent opposites had attracted. Audrey has always been an insulated, no-nonsense artist. Well, all art is artificial, etcetera, and the minute you interpret nature, the less likely that you remain a part of it. The garden I worked in was the perfect example. It was the unlikeliest combination of Rousseau and Léger.

I started learning about painters as well as sculptors at Audrey's work sessions and Gene's atelier—especially at his Friday open house to which I was now welcome. These times at Gene's were really sophisticated; everyone was so worldly. My transformation was nothing less than miraculous. I was a kid from Miami one day and a jet-set intellect in the midst of earthshaking matters the next.

Those Fridays were something. Theories, dogmas, presumptions flew in and out the doors and windows like fireflies that spark and sputter and rarely illuminate anything but themselves. Still, the agitation and the glitter of these creatures and their acceptance of me in their midst made me feel I was no longer a lonely straggler but part of a family. I loved it. I was dumbfounded at how much I didn't know. I was breathless with all the things I heard, and knew I would have to learn, if I were to hold my own and be part of this larger world.

Listening carefully, I would not only get the gist of what was happening in New York or Paris or San Francisco but would plan to show off my newfound knowledge the following day. No dice. A booming voice would contradict everything just uttered and I had only a choice of echoes. I mean, I had to use my noodle. I started to think at Gene Massin's, and because of him.

When I'd quit college and my future became cloudy, a terrible thing occurred to me. How would I carry my own weight, disabled and vulnerable as I was? How was I going to bring home the bacon? "Do you know what your mother and I expect and want your job to be right now? Staying as healthy as you can. That's your job." What a career I'd devoted myself to. I was working toward a gold watch and an office party.

During this Gene Massin-Audrey Wright period, I first considered and started planning a life that wasn't beyond my capacities. This time I wasn't dreaming up an impractical calling, but a genuine outlet for urges and propensities I'd observed all my life. The world of aesthetics in general—of sculpture in particular—along with all the accompanying, marvelous bullshit, was for me. The fraternal life of the artist was warming and helped awaken

146

me to this glorious fact. Polishing the gift I was given along with a crummy pancreas, I could express my feelings positively and to some possible advantage to others as well. By abstracting my anguish, I could lessen the pain and carve it into a shape more acceptable to others. When I later came to recognize my own anger as well, I could even release that with sometimes happy and even permanent result.

It hit me that the world was not made up entirely of Miami, the Rice House, doctors, the Foundation and myself. There was an astonishing prospect from the top of Gary Kleiman, and for the first time I used what was left of my eye to enjoy the view.

Forgettable as most of the discussions were those Fridays, I became aware that ideas, assailable as they might be, could prevail and conquer. Ideas acted upon were rays of light in the darkness. Passions could be roused by something other than pain and sex. Caught, on one of those Fridays, in the crossfire between antagonists brandishing their paintbrushes and carving tools, one would have thought they were fighting over a woman. Work and fulfillment meant so much to these people, more, it seemed, than fame and comfort. They were really alive.

I was romantic at twenty and, as with everything else in my life, incurable. I loved it all at Gene's—especially the companionship, the noise, the action. I'd get so excited by all the marvelous rapping that I'd have to sneak off and adjust my food and insulin intake, praying that nobody noticed. This was all so much more engrossing than my fucking numbers game. As for sex as a topic of diversion, it commanded about as much discretion and shamefaced propriety as a Claes Oldenburg-er.

Interestingly enough, straitlaced Marge and Marty Kleiman approved of my new involvements, grateful for my fresh animation. No matter what my mother might have thought of the condition of all the houses she delivered me to, she refrained from cleaning them and said nothing.

If first Gene Massin and then Audrey Wright opened up new worlds to me—worlds of mental gymnastics and work disciplines—then my next step was the biggest. I had learned to question and invent answers when I couldn't find them; and then I'd learned the pleasure of creating, of setting myself a task and following through. Whether through the kitchen door or not, I had entered the art world and I will always be grateful. But nothing prepared me, not even her son, Rod, for Edna Glaubman.

Edna was a local artist, a lovely painter who was beautiful, bright, gifted and insightful. She had a beauty mark and a husband, Maury, who looked like a thin Orson Welles and managed her career. At the time, she was doing vertical, batiklike abstractions in browns, blacks and whites. Very nice. Her palette has brightened since, become more vivid—Balinese in quality. But Edna was vivid from the start. Strong, direct, rhapsodic, she and her household, where I found another haven, were blessedly undisciplined. As at Gene's, the talk was endless, but here the warmth was penetrating.

On that first day that Robin picked me up at Audrey's and took me to the Glaubman house, I voyaged down the rabbit hole. There was no time at Edna's. No clock, no limits, no holds barred. No. There was a flow of life that carried everybody along, me included. There were lots of interruptions, mostly Mount Edna erupting beneficently, laughing hoarsely, putting herself and you on the line.

There was absolutely no shit countenanced at Edna's. Unlike admirers, TV people, congressmen and family, she would not be seduced or intimidated by my illness, or my tender age. She always addressed the human being.

When I got lugubrious and in the bluest of funks, commanding the stage with an announcement that I had had it, that another hemorrhage or reaction or a tarot card reading or just a momentary lack of resilience had made me decide to *quit*, to throw in the towel once and for all, Edna—who had plenty of her own troubles—shrugged her shoulders and said, "So quit. Go ahead and quit. Good-bye and good luck. Just do it and don't bore us all with talk about it."

I hadn't expected that reaction. There was no precedent for it

148

and it was a therapeutic kick in the ass. I thought it over later and decided it was great. Her impatience assumed a maturity and a basic health, attributes I craved. If I was going to falter or dramatize, I'd better get my act together. I, who was claiming to hate pity, should not be soliciting it. Everything had to be on my terms. Well, not with Edna Glaubman. She'd have none of that. Nonplussed though I was, I knew that people didn't talk turkey unless they really cared. Jesus, how I love no shit! At Edna's, everything came from the gut, and I got the warmth and emotional responses that replaced the sentimental reflexes I usually evoked. We had a lovely relationship, Edna and I.

Her son, Rod, my good friend, was a terrific musician, played a great guitar and, like his mother, was right on. "We are not playing chess, Gary," he would say to me when I parried, evaded or played dumb during a heavy conversation. "We're supposed to be talking so—let's *talk*—do you know what I mean?—talk, *communicate*. I'm over here."

Edna and Maury had another son, who had been crippled years before in a car wreck. He was in such a monstrous, dribbling, spastic state that I could only consider myself lucky to be me. Michael loved to hear his big, bearded brother make music, and quite unbelievably would occasionally laugh when some simple sensation would evidently delight him. Usually rebellious and impudent with authority figures—monuments I could scrawl my initials or some wicked graffiti on—I was always, from my earliest years, a sucker for kids or people who were as vulnerable as I. I loved making Michael laugh, and spent time with him, all the while thinking, *On my left is an endless line of people better off than I am and on my right, an endless line far worse. Where do I fit in?*

It was true that at Gene Massin's I learned to draw and think. At Audrey Wright's I learned technique and taste. It was at Edna Glaubman's that I developed perspective.

This was really bohemia, unboundaried, no longer even on the map. There are no longer any rules to bend. But then, back in 1973, I blossomed in this atmosphere. "Anything goes" should have been the password. It was the greatest—especially the give and take.

On my first visit to Edna's, I had just finished a small whale's tooth carving which I was polishing for sale. Edna loved it and wanted it.

"Will you give it to me?" she asked sweetly.

It was wild.

"Well, it's been promised."

"So what? I adore it. No one will adore it as much as I do no matter how they adore it."

I was flattered. I admired her work, and this approbation was coming not from my family but a real live "original" painter—a pro. She kept staring at the piece—a tiny abstract form that Audrey, too, had been pleased with.

"You were studying the duet on the wall in the next room. The painting of the cellist and pianist. Do you like it?"

"It's wonderful. You can hear the music."

"What are they playing?"

"A little something—very remote—by Wolfgang Amadeus Beethoven."

"How about us swapping?"

"You're kidding. What do you mean?"

"Do you know what swapping is? You take the painting, I get the carving."

"But that's not a swap. It's not a fair exchange. This is a little tiny—one of my first things—and the picture is immense and great and took so much more work and—"

"The first thing you've got to learn, Gary Kleiman, is to take a great offer when you get one."

"But—"

"Stop being ridiculous. So you're coming out ahead. Isn't that terrific? Good. It's a deal."

That lovely painting hangs in our house on North Bay Road, evidence of Edna's talent and utter indifference to conventional values. Both of these qualities made it essential that Maury supervise not only her business affairs but Michael's care as well.

Edna was so loving and free form that she could have organized a game of charades and put Michael on one of the teams. Whatever, his momentary needs were always satisfied, and despite her pain, she lived with his condition (until he died recently), as she did the changeable weather. She sort of didn't acknowledge illness, and in not bugging me at all she became a permissive, surrogate mother.

Robin couldn't believe my attachment to this family or the time I spent with them. Theirs was an even more unconventional ambience than Gene Massin's, which had disturbed her. An "original" was always showing up to say or do what I still believed to be original things. Robin found it all to exotic for comfort. The artist's life was not for her, and she thought my new interests were obviously dividing us. What she should have realized was that Edna understood me and was actually her ally and not mine.

"Gak!" Edna bellowed in her whiskey contralto. "You are a total fraud. You're always begging people to come nearer, nearer, *nearer*—"

"So?"

"So, wow, when we do, you turn on that red light so fast. Not even amber. No warning at all. Just stop! Crash! Bang! What a phony."

What an epitaph.

# 18

"**D**O YOU BELIEVE IN fate?" Judie asked me. She has just entered my life and at the eleventh hour.

"Yes," I answered, obviously impressed by the timing. "But I don't want to relinquish control. I mean, I believe, have to believe, that I have *some* say in the matter. What about you? Do you believe in fate?"

"When it's convenient," she replied.

She's really great for me, and I pray I won't screw it up. You see, she lives in town. I'm trying to turn over a new leaf, so let's see what's happened when we get to page 250.

My creatinine count doesn't seem to want to go below about 1.8 and often rises to two and over which is not good. The Cyclosporin has been reduced to a minimum and just when we feel we've really reached a balance and everything seems stabilized, whamm!

I just had to move my ass. Since my beautiful pal Debbie Seigler, a colleague at the hospital was in North Carolina and wanted to really go north, I flew up and we both went to see Glenn and Gise in Hartford, visited Newport, and just wandered around the Big Apple. It was just a weekend and I'm back at the diabetes unit and the Children's Diabetic Clinic at Fort Lauderdale. How I recognize—no matter their age or temperament—that unmistakable stamp of resentment and disbelief. *Why did this happen to me?* And *If I deny the whole business it will go away.* And yet—they are not at the clinic only because their families have brought them. Ambivalence is the key word. *I may save myself from coma and shock by being here and maybe they'll tell me it's all been a big mistake and I'll never have to take care of myself again. How can I admit I didn't keep the necessary records of my progress? Maybe he'll make me do it and I'll be OK.*

I saw Rinaldo, one of my patients, this morning. He's about twenty and he walked into my office early. He was sheepish as he said, "Gary, I have a friend down home in Bolivia who has diabetes, too. And he ain't taking care of himself. Can he have terrible things happen? You know, he eats the wrong things and he don't watch his urine like you said you gotta. Will it matter so bad that he can die or something terrible?"

Apparently, Rinaldo had been listening carefully at our previous meetings. He'd absorbed information about the severity of this disease that accepts no excuses. But perhaps not enough.

"Rinaldo, I can see you're worried about your friend. Does he see a doctor in Bolivia?"

"Yes. But he won't listen."

"What seems to be his biggest problem?"

"He just forgets to test. And he says the other guys are having Cokes and ice cream and things and he don't want to feel different."

"I remember you used to say you felt different, too."

"Yeah." But his eyes lowered.

"What made you begin to change, to feel OK about it?"

"I was tired of lying to my family and to you—and I couldn't remember the lies too good."

We both laughed.

"You made me realize that when I did good, I felt good. It was a good different."

I had to remember that I was talking to Rinaldo through his "friend."

"And your friend in Bolivia doesn't feel good or proud of himself now?"

153

"No."

"What would you like to tell this friend, Rinaldo?"

"To *do* it," he almost shouted.

We laughed again. But I thought, *How can I encourage him?*

"How do you think you can manage that? How can you convince him?"

This time, Rinaldo's eyes lighted up. "Maybe like the time when you made me feel good about some of *my* dumb things by telling me about squirting it in your mouth and going in the boat all day."

When I was nine, I swallowed my insulin one morning so I wouldn't have to shoot myself. I thought it would work. From both the effect and lack of it, it did not. He was also remembering that at day camp as a boy, I wanted to prove I was healthy and took a long canoeing trip without food and medication. Denial. Denial. Like Rinaldo's "friend."

"That's a good idea, Rinaldo. If it worked for *you*, then—"

"Yeah. It did, but I was worried a little. Anyway, I brought in real good records this week, see?" he added brightly.

And the records were meticulous. I wondered why he was guilty, unless he hadn't followed his meal plan. Was he testing me or himself?

They lumber into the clinic with the weight of this fucking disease dragging them down and no one can lift the burden. We can only help them to become strong enough to bear it.

Rinaldo slicked down his hair with the palm of his hand and shyly smiled good-bye as little Chicuco sidled in with his mother. Chicuco is twelve years old, his mother not much older. He's an intelligent kid, but already a master of denial. The pattern is classic. He's not only lazy about balancing his diet but sees no reason to. He won't accept the diagnosis and doesn't know why he's being dragged from a baseball game by Mrs. Palomo, who is his Marge. He is embarrassed, because it's hardly macho to be towed places by your mother, especially to a clinic, which in his mind brands him *sick*, to discuss this thing that isn't even visible and hasn't been discernible except maybe *sometimes*.

154

He used to wet his bed until he started taking insulin. This brought some kind of management to this first stage of diabetes. His symptoms have not yet reached their grisly diversity. He does take his insulin, so what do we all want from him? Simple. I want to do for him what no one did for me. I, too, did the minimum, and only to avoid nausea or worse. He can't conceive the potential.

Mrs. Palomo speaks barely a word of English, but is wildly communicative. She is as lively and concerned as Chicuco is bored and removed. As I talk with him, he plays with his Rubik's cube, even referring to a little pamphlet every once in a while. He'll look at anything except straight at me.

"I test, Gary. I swear it," he mumbles.

"*Es verdad!*" his mother agrees enthusiastically in the hope that my believing him will be the cure-all.

The boy is charming even when he makes no effort, and he's making no effort now. The constant shrug of his shoulder in response to my simple questions begins to look like a tic. He just refuses to be reached this session; but, in fierce competition with the Rubik's cube, I keep trying.

"I think, Chicuco, that your biggest trouble is with your shoulders. You're going to strike out if you keep bouncing them around." This was too confusing for Mrs. Palomo to decipher, but Chicuco begrudgingly smiled.

"Do you remember why we take insulin?"

"To help the sugar."

"Right. To help the sugar. They've got to go together. Remember the school dance? You've got to go with somebody. The sugar when it goes into your system has to have an escort, like your sister, Concepcion. You know. She can't go alone. The insulin is her date. If the cake and ice cream or whatever go to the dance without the insulin as escort, there are two bouncers—two strong-arm guys, like policemen—they're the kidneys—and they throw the sugar out on its butt and it's bounced into the urine. Get it?"

"Yep!"

"Where is it bounced into, Chicuco?"

"It gets bounced into the urine."

"Right. But what happens if the sugars are escorted by insulin?"

"They can stay at the dance."

"Right. One can't stay without the other. Now, if you take the insulin but you don't have the right amount or right type of food, you're kicked out of the gym another way. The guys with no date scream for a partner and then there's the *reaction*. Instead of dancing the body starts to shake for food."

Chicuco speaks English, but I might as well be talking to his mother, who gets one word in fifty although she gamely makes the most of each one. She eagerly smiles her corroboration of anything I might be saying, because she is in a hospital with a sick son and I am, to her, if not to the AMA, the doctor and may help him. I pause with some impatience because I'm not getting through today, and the kid looks up from his multicolored problem to see what I'm up to as he twists and turns the toy.

I touched his shoulder. "I know what a drag it is to keep testing, but this is the only way to really know what's happening. I want you to have a lot of energy for baseball."

"*Bahsebahl,*" Mrs. Palomo repeated gaily, intent on making this a pleasant visit and sensing a need for positivity.

Suddenly, the kid looked me squarely in the wrong eye. I was startled by the direct, candid right on, one on one look he threw me.

"You have diabetes too, don't you?"

"Yes."

"Is it true that your eyes are broken?"

I don't know where he heard this. It certainly isn't that obvious but I now thought I understood his refusal to get into focus. His tone was almost accusing.

"Yes, Chicuco."

"Can they be fixed?" he asked.

"I'm afraid not."

And then he asked it.

"They get broken because of diabetes, didn't they?"

That question and the need to answer it jolted me back to the past. I had asked all the same questions and had been given no answers—just sweet evasions, euphemisms or what turned out to be deceit. I believed them all. I wanted to believe. I collaborated. I had been given the little hope that was the lie. But diabetics mature as well as age quickly. Jesus! We *have* to know the truth.

"Not everybody with diabetes gets this, Chicuco. There are no guarantees but you've got to remember that when I got diabetes back in 1960 you weren't even born and things are very different in 1983. We've gone to the moon, for Christ's sake. The insulin is purer and all the tests are much more exact. *If you test!* They've learned so much and, Chicuco, I *didn't* take care of myself sometimes. I lied and got bored and I always thought my mother was bugging me."

*Oh God, Chicuco, listen, you crazy kid!*

Chicuco was startled, then with shining eyes he looked at his mother for the first time with something that approached tenderness and the sweet lady picked up the cue fast if inaccurately.

"Bugging me!" she said, nodding in delight. "*Sí. Sí.* Bugging me." Obviously the examination was going well.

"*Oye, Mamacita!*" Both the kid and I were now laughing.

"Yes, Chicuco, I did a lot of wrong things. Anyway, the bottom line is signed by you. *You're* the boss."

I was all over the joint, playing all sides. He had to know that first he had a problem and it wasn't the mumps. Second, that even the mumps can be a problem, and third, that no matter what he had, there was a way of handling and possibly beating it.

No matter how young my patients may be, I always try to return some of the self-importance they had before they were zapped by things out of their control. Because they are forced to diet and take medicine daily, they have lost their most precious possession—freedom. Since they must comply with the rules of the game of war against diabetes, the counselor, doctor, parent or guardian must repay the child in the best coin possible. If the diabetic child can no longer have his freedom, then he must be allowed and encouraged to be his own keeper. It sounds unrealistic. It is not. I know. A child must and can be made to be in charge of himself and do *more* than what the doctor has ordered. He must be respected and trusted as the doctor's partner and then eventually be trained to be his own savior.

I try to find the character in the child and then help develop it. It's ticklish, it's delicate, but it's thrilling to see children use their newfound sovereignty to their own advantage. Certainly there will be backslides and some resistance, but with the counselor's and clinician's patience and empathy eventually they will exercise their own discipline with pride. But you've got to make them tough after you've soothed them. "Quality in everything and quality must be tested." It's true, but along with Woody Allen in *Love and Death*, I wish instead I could have taken a written!

All diseases have their MO. Not so with this little bugger. Except for the dramatic loss of weight that usually accompanies uncontrolled diabetes, there is little visible evidence of diabetes's existence. My appearance and general demeanor, my energy level, all give the lie to the facts. It's like Disney World. Smooth and easy, but it's all showmanship, with the effort and sweat underground. I love it. The facade allows me to be more successful with the kids. With a lot of horsing around thrown in, we can talk of our common burden without frightening the hell out of them.

We've got to mold constructive fear that brings prudence out of the chaos of the diabetics' bewilderment. Once more, it's the delicate balance. I want the kids to have the fear that cautions against danger, makes them smell it. This fear is designed and encouraged to save their lives. What we must do, however, is to avoid creating the unselective fear that restricts and paralyzes.

There is always the quality of life to be considered, along with simple survival. And so—at the clinic, everywhere—with kids, we show them the best and worst probabilities and give them the possibility of determining their own futures. That sense of power is vital. I know this much for sure. Medical people who seduce patients with false hope should be brought up on some kind of

158

psychical rape charge. The poisoned fruit of such a relationship is far more ravaging than the control systems that must be immediately set up and confirmed as valuable by any active, long-term diabetic counselor. Anyway, it's the best we can do without a cure. Maybe the kids, if they really like us, will use us as models.

At twenty, instead of allowing myself to be chipped away, I decided to use my own tools to model myself after others, and I started to study and to work and carve my own future, such as it was.

# 19

WHAT COULD BE MORE God-like than creating form, giving life to clay, design and order to stone and metal and then to yourself? Having no authority to reshape my past, I experienced a surge of power as I worked with Audrey and first felt the thrill of even clumsy creation. I became obsessed with work and barely slept. I was engaged all day at Audrey's and then at night I labored in a makeshift studio on the side of our house on Palm Island. My parents had fixed up a sort of guesthouse for me and it couldn't have been better, suiting me just fine. Chips and pulverized stone and plaster dust were everywhere, and I felt a proper artist.

Absolutely driven, I would work until three or four in the morning or until Marge, the night watchman, seeing the light from her bedroom window, would call, begging me to pack it in. I would mumble something like "Artists don't need to sleep," and in a half hour or so, in self-satisfied fatigue, I'd go to my room, do my testing and fall asleep, only to be up at seven-thirty so Marge could drop me off at Audrey's by nine. Sick or well, I could still do that at twenty.

This was every night. I was serious and I was having a ball. Completing at least one piece a week, I was selling them to friends who might have been trying to encourage me but seemed to like them as well. I think they got their money's worth. Anyway, my energy level was manic.

One day, suffering from another hemorrhage, I was out of commission and Audrey came to my place for a change. She claimed she was just passing by. Yeah! Slapping a piece of plaster in my hand—I remember, it felt like a paper cup in shape—she said, "You carve it like this." She carefully handed me the handle of a knife and guided my hand as we cut a slot through the middle of it.

"Now, go on from there. Play with it."

Bleeding and sightless, I did as I was told, and, damnit, if at the end of the day I didn't feel the shape of a horse that had me galloping through another crisis.

For a few years, I was to have those terrible hemorrhages everywhere, at home, up north, in England. They were a torment and eventually a bloody bore. I waited, helpless, since the eyes could not be treated until the blood disappeared. Both Dr. Norton and Dr. George Blankenship at Bascom Palmer had to time their laser treatments perfectly and did. My concerned questions were now becoming more sophisticated as I unfortunately was becoming a pro. The answers, by necessity, were more detailed: I had to know everything and they informed me, trying always to hold out a grain of hope without resorting to deceit.

"Is there any change for the good, Doctor?" I asked Dr. Norton.

"There's no such thing, Gary, in your case. Only the impossible reversal. All change is further deterioration. It's *no* change we are looking for."

He couldn't have made it clearer. Then I would get the good news.

"But everything beside the bleeding is stable."

In my case, I was to learn that the hemorrhages themselves were simply symptomatic and not determining factors. It was the curative laser treatments that were unavoidably and further destroying my vision. The blood, I was to recognize, would always eventually subside, receding like the sea from the beach.

And so I got used to the damned things, conserving my energy for the long haul, leaving me with virtually the same bit of vision undisturbed. I got less frightened, too, and eventually, a couple of years ago, the hemorrhages stopped. I'd gotten to know my demons so well, they had become so predictable, that they had to start planning new surprises.

Diabetic or not, I was an artist now and decided to move to the artists' colony in Coconut Grove. Lucky enough to have had a trust fund set up for me that was supposed to be available when I graduated from college or got married, I was allowed to invade the trust at this time, since both those conditions seemed unlikely.

I wanted to be like Audrey and Gene and I bought the first place that turned up—a tiny, wonderful house all my own. A place I could be completely myself in and mess up with all the junk I owned and all the plaster and residue of my trade. Without my mother's admonishments to force me into order, I found my own inherited compulsions replaced hers. The minute I moved in I became fastidious. I carpeted, bought track lighting, some good pictures, some nice, simple furniture, and there was only one thing missing.

Since I was rushing headlong from my innocent teens into the sophisticated half-world of the Left Bank, and after not even calling her for three weeks, I asked Robin to live with me. It was my shrewdest mistake.

I couldn't lose. If she accepted, I had a healthy, really sharp, mature, new image. If she refused, I would be free to commit myself to me exclusively. You know, my career! It's lonely at the top! He travels fastest, etcetera!

Of course, Robin rejected the idea out of hand. She thought I was demented as well as highly neurotic. My aggressive, indelicate offer only confirmed her suspicions about my degenerate friends and their influence on me. My invitation killed our ailing romance. It was no surprise. I was too much of a handful for her—and everybody else.

My damned-up energy was spilling and leaking and about to flood the Left Bank. For someone who had always sought mischief and pleasure, I was now trying to express another part of me

162

still undefinable. I know only that this was the beginning of my race against time.

I was making appearances for both the Foundation and Dr. Mintz, who was having those spectacular beta cell results with rats. If only I had been a rat. If I couldn't, then I could die some kind of artist instead of an ailing clown.

Thumbing through art books was difficult—my desire to study had come too late—so I flew up to New York and Washington and stood before great works. I haunted museums and galleries, and when I returned I asked Audrey who she thought was the greatest sculptor in the country. She never even paused.

"Isamu Noguchi," she said.

"He doesn't sound American," the fledgling replied.

There were so many blanks to fill in. I had seen a lot up north, but my vision was pretty concentrated.

If Noguchi was the best, I had to examine him carefully.

When I first saw his work, I spaced out. Talk about revelation! It was like looking up at the sky and seeing another moon or something. One after another, his work had a profound effect on me. *MU*, the Greek marble; *Black Sun in Granite* and the bronze *Mytosis*—which sounded like something I'd eventually develop—the gray marble *In Silence Moving* and the exquisite white Carrara marble *Integral*. I had never seen shapes like that. And then his versatility—the playgrounds, gardens, landscapes, stage sets. Unbelievable!

I had to meet this guy. I was really studying up on my craft, ogling everything I could get my hands on for fear that at any time I could lose the rest of my sight. But no one affected me up to that moment like Noguchi. I mean it when I say I was spaced out. Since this was the space age, I was going to move light-years ahead and reach him, not by telescope but rocket.

I flew to New York with slides of my work, all my medications and gall that could have been divided in three parts. I couldn't be alive at the same time as this genius without meeting him. Maybe some of the moonglow would rub off. Maybe I could learn the secret of creation. After all, it was the opposite of disease and death. My astonishment was boundless and could have carried me to New York without Eastern's 727, which my parents thought more practical.

He was not waiting at the airport, and I had no idea where to find him. I went to the Museum of Modern Art and some bright person behind the information desk said, "Who is he?"

"One of the guards," I answered. "I'm a lawyer here to inform him that he has come into a great inheritance."

I then went to the Whitney and Guggenheim museums, who had heard of him but couldn't give me his number. It never occurred to me to look in the New York telephone book—not even in the Yellow Pages under G for genius—the simple directory, but there he was. *Noguchi, Isamu.* That brilliant teacher back in third grade had been right after all. "Just look under N." He was just there, like fresh air, not hidden but available to anyone.

Tracking him down through the all-knowing Ma Bell, I got his studio and talked with his charming secretary, Melody Sternoff, who had previously been associated with Priscilla Morgan of the Spoleto festivals. Noguchi was not in New York but in Italy. I was to be kept in suspense for a couple of months, but I presented my credentials, not hesitating to tell my whole story. God knows, there had to be *some* advantages accruing.

Miss Sternoff couldn't have been more sympathetic. She was certain that the sculptor would be glad to meet with me when he returned. Back in Florida, after catching up on some more of his pieces, I wrote to him of my admiration and my dreams. I also sent an article about me that had just been published in Miami.

I must say that Noguchi is, like his work, surrounded by space. He may be in the Manhattan phone book, but your minute is up all too quickly. He has his eye on his assured immortality. And still, he answered my petition as honestly as I'd written it. I recall fragments. "I am a lonely traveler and no source of comfort, I fear. . . . I am distressed at your troubles and understand your need for proof of your existence . . . work is that only proof. . . . I know that I must leave as much as possible as evi-

164

dence of *my* brief stay. . . . I may not be in New York, but do not say I won't be in New York . . . I should love to meet you and maybe in October, if I'm back from Japan. . . ."

When summer was over, Glenn and I went up to New York to visit our Aunt Tobia and see the sights. New York is always great in the fall and the heat was on back home. Of course, I had one sight in mind. I called Noguchi's studio and spoke to Melody, who informed me that he was very much in town and if I wished to call him, she would give me his home number.

It was a Wednesday and he was on the wire, electrifying me. It had been so easy, really. Why do people make things so difficult for themselves? "I would love to meet with you, Noguchi," I heard myself say. Since he was always called Noguchi by everyone, I thoughtlessly addressed him that way. I mean, I was such a moron. It's a wonder I didn't say, "Kleiman at this end!" But he seemed not to be offended. It would take more than protocol to ruffle him. As a matter of fact, I can't think of anyone saying Mr. Picasso or Mr. Buonarroti. Maybe! But I was talking to a legend. The legend now said, "Why don't you meet me at my apartment and we'll drive to my studio together."

"That would be great!"

"What about Friday?"

On Friday morning, right on time, Glenn and I arrived at his apartment, but the doorman was unimpressed first by our punctuality and then by our presence altogether. Noguchi was not at home.

"But he's expecting us," I insisted.

"He is *not* at home," was the accusing response.

One would have thought Glenn and I were hoods trying to ransack the place. Glenn was embarrassed by the situation and was ready to slink off. I couldn't believe what was happening.

"I don't understand," I went on. "We were asked to be here and I've come a long way—"

And then a slim, lovely girl with immense eyes materialized at the entrance.

"You must be Gary Kleiman!"

"Yes. This is my brother, Glenn."

"Hello. I'm Melody Sternoff. What's the trouble? We're all supposed to drive out to Long Island City together. It's all right, Jimmy. We're expected."

Well, his secretary was as mystified as I until with further investigation she discovered that Noguchi was in Flower Hospital on Fifth Avenue, for something so vague that it had no name. We got the impression that it was simply a need of rest and quiet. Glenn wondered with a glint whether it wasn't a rather elaborate way of avoiding me.

Melody, who should never have been called Sternoff, which sounded like a reprimand, was as lovely as her given name. After sorting things out, she invited us to come to the studio with her and she would then try to arrange a future appointment.

When we entered Noguchi's old, Long Island City studio, the first work I saw was the white Carrara marble *Integral* I had fallen for. It was patiently lying on its side, having a scratch repaired. It was a moment of sweetest intimacy for me. At the risk of sounding like a believer, I thought I'd entered heaven. My next encounter was with the gray marble *In Silence Moving*, which stood gracefully, almost demurely, catching the light.

There was a maze of small rooms filled with work—mostly unknown to me—some sketches, studies, masterpieces. The body of work there in the studio made my fingers itch. Melody took us through what looked like a heavy bolted barn door where there was a small kitchen, a table, chairs, a cot and lots of books. A staircase led to a second floor you couldn't enter without discarding shoes and all preconceived notions of what a pad should look like. I had just created my own setting, but this was thirteen steps to Kyoto. The peace and beauty were all-pervasive, like the delicate scent of flowers. The rice-paper walls and cardboard rolls across the ceiling, the diffused lighting and alabaster carvings all seemed to melt one into the other, creating a calm and endless horizon within a relatively small space.

"Wow!"

166

"It's lovely, isn't it?" Melody asked.

Glenn was speechless. That's tough for me.

"What a place to dream, to hang around."

"There isn't too much of that going on, here. Let's see your slides. You promised to show them to us."

Melody was generous in her appraisal of my work. And I knew she was sincere, because she left to call Noguchi; she told him of my great disappointment and asked if he would see me at the hospital. He agreed, and a few days later I went to Flower Fifth.

There are moments when I am overwhelmingly grateful for my speck of vision. With beautiful women, sunsets, works of art, remarkable human beings. I was thankful that I could *see* Noguchi, uncharacteristic as his repose was that day. Spare and wiry, even prone he moved like electricity. Like his work, there was nothing excessive in his design. Even in bed he seemed in a divine hurry—like you know who—only he's always late for a date with his muse and not his jester.

I was subsequently to see him as the dervish he is, but that day in the hospital, he looked really cute lying in bed being fed with chopsticks out of a perfect, little blue bowl by a pretty Japanese.

If anyone has ever been, in art and life, the bridge that spans east and west, it is Isamu Noguchi. I marveled at his golden, strong hands—they really looked golden—and his striking blue eyes, a gift from his mother and the rest of the Gilmours. He is of and beyond both worlds.

He studied my slides, and we sat in silence, my heart pounding. I had adjusted my insulin and food intake to absorb the meeting.

"How long have you been working?"

"About five months."

He sighed. His voice became wistful.

"Sometimes it's best not to become too successful."

"You mean, not too soon?"

"No! I mean sometimes not at all."

I had carved another whale ivory abstraction and dared present him with it.

"Yes, Brancusi said, 'When an artist stopped being a child, he stopped being an artist.'"

I found his words encouraging and mysterious.

"Use what's in your area, Gary. In Florida, coral rock is good. It's brittle, but it can be carved."

Prepared for my moment in history, I had brought his biography with me. I now asked him if he would inscribe it as a gift to my teacher. He did, after a moment's thought.

> Gary speaks of Audrey
> To whom he takes this book
> Audrey finds Gary
> And Gary finds the world
> —*Isamu Noguchi*

Then, in his most reasonable and imperial manner, he evicted me. He'd had it. He sliced a farewell through the air with his hand and dispensed with me.

"There's an excellent exhibition at the Guggenheim. See it."

And so the first of many meetings was at an end.

Flying home to Florida, I was carving shapes in the sky, using the plane as a tool. I know I sound like instant coffee or something, but I felt, after selling a lot of little figures, that I was really ready—if not for the big time, for bigger things. I was impatient for the next step, and my little house, which I now imagined with its graphics and plaster dust was a real live atelier, became both my stage and my prison.

# 20

**M**UCH AS I LOVED sculpting, I hated being alone. Dependent on my family or friends to get around, I prayed, as the saying goes, for telegrams. I could work fifteen straight hours with other students, but after two at home, I would have welcomed a second-story man for company. Unlike my idols, I could never be too removed from people. If I could have set up shop in the middle of the Orange Bowl, Wimbledon or Times Square, I would never have stopped working. If I could have shared a Tab or an apple with a chum every once in a while and heard the screeching brakes and honking horns of human relations, there would have been no end to my produce. No matter how homey my workshop was, I couldn't leave it at will. That makes any place a prison.

I even rented a room out for a while to a guy about forty who had just been divorced, but we were the odd couple and that was that. I sometimes wondered whether I'd invited Robin to share my new life because I needed a roommate. Only Dylan remained faithfully by my side, but he wasn't into great conversation and, worse yet, he couldn't drive. He certainly understood and deplored my needs. Every time the telephone would ring, he knew I'd soon be off and he'd be alone. I guess it's something a lot of us avoid. He'd really glower at me. There was real reproach, even scorn. Boy, did he know me and did he hate that telephone. It was I who was being saved by the bell.

I believe I finished so many pieces so very quickly so that I could legitimately go have them based. That was where the action was. Outside. It was never lonely at Audrey's or at the Massins'.

I was casting my work now—in bronze—and was still shocked that I was actually receiving silver for it. I had been struck dumb when the first person asked how much I wanted for my work. I was suspicious that it was charity, a possibility I had found sickening. I was never certain that anyone was buying my work because he liked it. This has been a continuing torture. The only times I have been at peace with this have been those in which the buyers were totally unaware of my problem.

Still, with all the action, there must have been a lingering resentment that my youth had been stolen; and I would simply pick up and go to Gainesville to see friends at the University of Florida.

On one particular junket, an old tennis buddy drove me up, and in the middle of a party I just got a feeling I was ready for bigger things. I called Noguchi in New York. I knew he'd be working at his studio. It was a most surprising conversation.

"I hope I'm not interrupting you, Isamu. This is Gary Kleiman."

"How are you, Gary?"

"Fine, thank you. And you?"

"Fine. Your work going well?"

"I think so. I'd like to enlarge some of my work. How do I go about it?"

"I don't do that sort of thing. I don't enlarge. I work big when I want. I think you should speak to Henry Moore."

I couldn't believe it. *I think you should speak to Henry Moore. Sure!*

"Thanks. Say hello to Melody and keep working, now. See you later." *I think you should speak to Henry Moore!* Well, why not?

I made a person-to-person call to the Marlborough Gallery in London and asked how I could reach Moore. I was calling from Gainesville, Florida, I said, on the suggestion of Isamu Noguchi,

170

and it was of great importance. England! The gallery politely gave me a number and in two seconds I was speaking with a gracious Mrs. Moore in Hertfordshire—in three with Henry Moore himself.

Life couldn't be tougher, but, Jesus, things can be so easy. It's like trouble with the phone company or the bank. Don't screw around with supervisors. Go to the top. The president of a corporation is too secure to be snide. He can afford to be accommodating, right? The top is accessible if you just don't wait for the elevator.

"Hello, hello! This is Henry Moore."

The voice was thin, reedy and so upper class that I was afraid he'd hang up when I spoke. I trotted out my terrible credentials.

"My name is Gary Kleiman."

I thought of Gene Massin, who always called me a TND—a top-notch diabetic! I had become a stand-up tragedian.

"I'm calling from Florida—America. I'm twenty-one, a sculptor and I've lost most of my sight—" That seemed to hook everybody. "I'd love to meet you and ask your advice. Isamu Noguchi suggested I call."

"Well, I'm off to Italy late in June for a spell of carving."

"Oh," I said, disappointed.

"If you can come before, that will be fine."

"I'll see you Sunday," I answered quickly.

"When you get to England, call and I shall give you directions."

I hung up, gave a giant hoot and started dialing.

"Hello. Hello, Dad?"

"Gar. How's everything?"

"Smashing, old top!"

"Are you having your reactions in dialect now?"

"Never mind the comedy. How would my pater, Sir Morty Kleinberg, like to go to England now that spring is here?"

"What's the deal?"

"I spoke to Noguchi about enlarging my work and he told me to get in touch with Moore—Henry Moore!"

"You've got to be kidding!"

"I just got off the phone. He invited us over. I told him we'd be there Sunday. Are you packed yet?"

"All but my London Fog."

"There'll be plenty of that when we get there!"

As the reader must know by now, my father has gone to hell and back for me, so why not beautiful England? When he suggested later that I go with a friend whose tab he'd pay, I refused. There was really no one as much fun to be with. Marge knew we were buddies and understood.

He and I could travel carefreely without reservations, laundry service and a religiously kept itinerary. She was concerned because of my recent setback but knew it would be useless to try dissuading me. At least with my father, she knew I'd be safe, especially since *he* knew London. She gave us her blessing, and then put on her act.

"Say hello to Elizabeth and Philip."

"What about Elizabeth and Richard?"

"Them, too."

"What about Elizabeth and Essex?" Marty asked.

I was waiting for the usual warnings. For someone who was always worried stiff about me, she was always stoically seeing me off to possible disaster every time the fancy struck me. I was now over twenty-one and something told her to beware. I still got the message even when she said, "If they're at all available, Gary will manage that, too."

"Not bad, Mom. You're getting the idea."

I had been giving my mother lessons in humor. You know, like "Tell your joke, don't hang around to explain it; say it and run and *don't laugh.*" She was really getting better. She didn't laugh or anything.

My father and I, without reservations, checked into a small hotel in Kensington—a sort of Sir Howard Johnson's. We had taken a midnight flight and, on arriving, had gone straight to bed. Aside from jet lag, I got all mixed up and took what I thought was my morning dose of insulin. Overcompensating for the time change, I went into hypoglycemic reaction. Earlier, the bellboy had told us that he would deliver our door key, which also fit an automatic food machine in our room, but we never heard from him again. This vendor was supposed to supplement or, I guess, substitute for room service, which this place had never heard of. I could see my mother's face. We had done everything wrong without her.

Awaking with a pounding headache an hour after retiring, I was now sweating thirty-two calibers, trembling, sick and in need of food. If Marge had been along, she calmly would have produced out of nowhere, or her purse, a five-course meal with precisely the proper balance of sugar, carbohydrates and protein with that infuriating assurance that prevented life's vagaries from ever finding her wanting.

"Dad, you'd better get me something fast."

We both were banging on the blasted machine. My emotional father, giving the unyielding monster one last punch, tried contacting room service and then went raving into the corridors to steal sugar cubes from discarded breakfast trays. While I called downstairs again and calmly said that "someone" there was diabetic and needed sugar and food quickly, Marty flew downstairs and depleted a buffet table in the dining room of all sorts of wild appetizers, returning just as management sent up two glasses of what seemed like pure glucose and lots of buttered scones.

After a rest, I bounced back, praying that all these tidbits wouldn't throw me into somogyi. The minute I knew I was OK, I called Moore. Not without some trepidation. Would he remember inviting me? If so, was he still so disposed? Or had he been just kind or, worse yet, just eager to get off the hook.

This time he answered the phone himself. He remembered. If I was coming up from London, then I must take the directions very carefully. Did I have a pencil and paper? I will never forget those directions. There was everything but the bread crumbs. I mean, he really gives directions. Like, "There's a brook there and you'll come to a willow tree, and five and a half yards—"

173

I swear, I loved it. And the names. It was great. Perry Green, Much Haddam, The Hoglands. "And when a little yellow bird with a black and gray beak—" No! I added that, but it was almost that.

We found the little hamlet in Hertfordshire and Marty got us to the front door, where lots of boots were neatly lined up against the frame. As we knocked, we wondered whether we were supposed to enter in our stockinged feet.

Irina Moore, the sculptor's wife, welcomed us warmly and led us through a lovely, formal garden—very English. But not so much as Mr. Moore, who was photographing an old piece cast in lead.

Henry Moore, then in his middle seventies, was a handsome man. Imposing, virile and aristocratic. His silvery head was wonderful, and though he was working he was neatly dressed, school tie and all. I'm sure he dresses to take a shower. Like Noguchi, he is preoccupied, but in a different manner. Both are totally involved with their work and would feel, in the presence of admirers, benefactors or detractors, a homesickness for their studios. I'm sure that, despite personal gratifications, they have the same loneliness *away* from their work that I have in the happy midst of it. I realized that I was—for all Moore's graciousness—an intruder, a phone call *he* had not been praying for.

Being Henry Moore is a career in itself, and with the help of his wife he must protect himself from his reputation. People come from all over the world—even from Miami—to touch greatness for a moment and maybe catch it like hepatitis. Or they come to worship at his shrine. It must be a bore for him after a while, that kind of adulation. Like the pope. You sense a weariness with such mass adoration.

Mr. Moore only had to be cued and he was off. He anticipated all of my questions and had his answers ready. He must repeat them over and over to the devoted. It was a familiar catechism—with one variation.

"Do you think," I asked, "that I could still do sculpture if I go totally blind?"

174

"You could, but it would be different. You would probably have to hand model, use clay first and then cast. Still, there are those who believe—along with the primitives—that that is the most creative of all."

"I'd love to show you my work," I said as I handed him my photos. My respect, at the moment, was equaled by my squeamishness as he now examined my work.

Nodding his head in what I hoped I interpreted correctly as some approval, he suddenly stopped at something I call *The Sprinter*. "I like this. I like this very much."

Imagine what I felt. Imagine a young painter being told by Picasso, who also wouldn't screw around, "*I like this.*" I mumbled something about my health and certain necessities and popped a Fig Newton into my mouth. He now rose and offered to show us his enlarging deck.

After covering a polystyrene working model in plaster, Moore then places grids over the whole thing. Through this network of horizontal and perpendicular lines—meticulously measured and spaced to locate points—all parts of the whole grow as a human child does, proportionately. In that great greenhouse flooded with daylight and through this grillage, Moore and his assistants can increase a work to any desired dimension. Good luck! With such mathematical prowess, I could have been an architect sitting at Buckminster Fuller's feet or a vet making Great Danes out of miniature poodles.

I really do, at times, acknowledge my limitations. Moore, sensing my despair, now gave me what I wanted—the name of his enlarger, Henraux, in Italy, whom he evidently used depending on the medium.

Mr. Moore couldn't have been less pressured and more generous with his time as he took us through his many studios and gardens. There were sculptures all over the joint. With breaks for elevenses and tiffin, this man worked from 8 A.M. to 7:30 P.M. He had his own date with destiny.

"I want to do as much work as possible in this lifetime."

Where had I heard that before?

175

We walked through his land, where grazing sheep sometimes nestled near his majestic figures, and he told me of his admiration for Cézanne. He loved reliefs of women's backs, like Cézanne. He loved women. Reclining women. Strong women. What's new? Tell me about it.

His favorite woman sculptor was Germaine Richier. He never mentioned Barbara Hepworth, whose work I had been told mine resembled. It was not an unlikely comparison since Audrey had emulated the English sculptor, and her influence must have seeped through to me.

And then, all three of us knew simultaneously that our visit was over. So different from Noguchi, who would have blue streaked it across the fields and told us to get lost in the National Gallery. A bell rings in Isamu's head and for the next round that's it for this world, and anyone in it. It's really great.

Moore sets great store in the vitality that bursts forth from the interior of all form, and it is his genius, I believe, that he conveys that life force in his work. But cute, dry, funny, abrupt, pure Noguchi—for me at least—evokes the spirit of things. He may tease you and in five minutes not know you're there, but when he is in contact, you fly. Warm and cold, sweet and sour, yin and Yank, he is finally not the bridge between east and west but the isthmus. I just love hanging around him.

Neither artist just hangs around, however. Of course, Isamu was, when first we met, in his feverish sixties, Moore in his scrupulous seventies. They are both going strong, still proving they've been here, still doing more.

When I told Edna Glaubman at one point that I had done thirty-four pieces, she said, "When you've stopped counting, I'll know you've done a lot of work."

# 21

I HAD NOW MET and profited from the two most renowned men of the world in which I had chosen to work. According to the men in white, I was already on velvet if not quilted satin. Greedy for life and wanting to be sure that there was "proof I'd been here," I was busy, but I wasn't satisfied.

Before leaving for Italy to see Mr. Moore's enlarger, Marty and I spent the afternoon at the Tate Gallery. The Blake pictures, the Michelangelo cartoon, the whole place was incredible, but Hepworth really turned me on. Everything in her work seemed to echo thoughts and feelings I had. It seemed strange, even with Audrey's pipeline, that I could feel this strongly about someone else's work. There was a kinship that I never felt with Moore or Noguchi, for all my awe and affection.

I asked questions. She wasn't young. She had been not too happily married to the sculptor-painter Ben Nicholson. Jesus, those two careers. Always remarkable, they had produced triplets. Barbara always gave it all she had.

I heard she was a difficult lady—with husband, with fellow sculptors, with Moore. With people who invaded her privacy. She was known to consent to an occasional interview and—before the first question was asked—dismiss the poor reporter out of hand, because of some gut reaction. I still wanted to meet her. I also had heard that she had a health problem, discreetly made vague by her and my informants. But there was an energy and love in her work and a certain, familiar something that drew me to her. It was said that among Brancusi, Moore, Noguchi and Hepworth, modern sculpture was created. I had to meet her. I had managed two out of the available three. Why not go for broke?

Not certain if I'd ever be in England again, I telephoned her in St. Ives from the Grosvenor Hotel, where we'd moved. I got somebody's number pronto. My father was still recovering from the experience of meeting Henry Moore. I think he would have preferred my quitting while I was ahead, but he ordered a double brandy while I put in my call to St. Ives.

I asked if I could speak with Dame Barbara Hepworth and she answered, "This is she." When I introduced myself, I now used Henry Moore as my entree. I had come to England to learn of enlarging. I had certain difficulties. I'm embarrassed to report the rest.

"Oh, my God!" Hepworth said with such genuine distress that I heard myself add, "It's OK. I mean, it's not that bad, really."

"Going blind isn't that bad—for a sculptor? Oh, my dear."

"It's all right. I live with it now. It's just that I admire your work and—"

But she was so shaken that I was sorry I'd mentioned my problem. It was a kind of open sesame, you know. I really hadn't anticipated such a heavy reaction.

"My father and I were at the Tate," I continued, "and when I saw your work I knew I had to meet you. I'm only in England for a few days more. Would it be possible?"

"Why, yes, my dear. Of course. Tuesday would be fine."

"Gee, I'm leaving Tuesday for France. Is Monday at all possible—please?"

There was a pause. She would change some appointments, and if I would not arrive any time before three, Monday would be fine.

178

"I'm in the center of this little town, Mr. Kleiman. Just ask anyone directions, you'll find me, I'm sure."

Marty and I had a wonderful drive down to this quaint seaside village somehow more like Portugal than England, and we stayed at a bed and breakfast place. We wandered through the picturesque town and walked the beach, and then at the dot of three we were met by Margaret Moir, Hepworth's secretary, who showed us through the place.

Again I was awed by the vast amount of visible work.

I was to be changed forever by our meeting. I have never seen a kinder nor a more radiant smile. When she wasn't smiling, her face was strong, perhaps ruthless, but when it grew soft, never have I had anyone look at me like that. She seemed to suffer another's pain and simultaneously relieve it. Her crinkly eyes saw and accepted everything.

Hepworth couldn't have been anything but a Brit and resembled, especially in profile, Queen Mother Elizabeth, with a little Julia Child thrown in. Although she used a three-pronged cane because of a hip injury, she seemed hearty and, when we greeted each other, the strength of her hand was alarming. Strength and tenderness, that was Barbara Hepworth. She was the holiest of my three big ones.

To Hepworth, the human spirit that she caught in her work inhabited everything, everywhere. She believed that the consciousness of man pervaded the landscape and all other forms of life.

Plagued by ill health, she still believed that all sculpture must be an act of praise and sensibility to the oneness of man and landscape. Looking into her face, I became ashamed. My landscape was filled with props to accompany my drama. My cluttered landscape up to then had been pretty circumscribed. Hers had no horizon.

I was so lucky to have been exposed even briefly to such people.

To be with the fugitive Noguchi was to be windswept, with Moore, majestically instructed from Olympus, with Barbara

Hepworth, to become part of the whole. I felt tranquil. I had never experienced tranquility before. I felt safe. I felt unlonely.

Her talk of the human figure, not separate from but part of the environment, sharpened my awareness even more, made me in a sense feel like a real creation myself. I can't help but observe that of all the media, common clay is the least durable. Nonetheless, I believe that though her sympathy with my plight was real and the accompanying tenderness the initial urge that suggested our friendship, it was my basic health that attracted her and sealed our bargain.

"Sculpture is an affirmative statement of our will to live."

That's what the lady said and I agree, although I fear I have never had the dedication, the ability to stand or sit alone in my quest for any real sustained period. But I've knelt and prayed at the altar of art and respect those who do. I love the idea, the concept, the goal, and then get on with it. I've yet to rise above my humanness as she did.

Starting with those Fridays at Gene Massin's, the happy intrusion of ideas into my life offered the long sufferer an alternate activity. It was called thinking, and though I came late to it, I really moved quickly from Huck's fence to Rodin's Gate of Hell. There was so much catching up to do.

I asked Hepworth what she thought of the possibilities of my continuing my work if the worst were to happen and my retina were completely destroyed.

She measured a distance in the air with both hands. "Do you know how much this is?"

"Yes."

She now extended the space. "And this?"

"Yes."

She smiled that enchanting smile. "Then you can work. You'll feel your way. You'll be fine."

Others had encouraged me, but when Hepworth said this, I knew nothing would stop me except Gary, the kid himself. Anyway, Hepworth drew and sculpted not what she literally saw but what she perceived. That, for Christ's sake, was art. That really gave me hope. After all, celebrated men and women of vision and insight were not being honored for twenty-twenty eyes.

"You must have been outraged when you found out about your eyes. The *injustice*; I would be *impossible*. When I was immobile for a while after an accident, I had to be in hospital and I could have burst. I was biting everyone's head off."

I believed every word of it.

Her companion, Jacquie Watson, brought us a very English tea with all the trimmings. I was more interested in Hepworth's reactions to my work; and I hung over her trying to translate her sighs and coughs and the tapping of her eternal cigarette as she chain-smoked.

Sensitive Barbara had a whole soundtrack going as she flipped the photos.

I was hearing civilized and rather upbeat "oh's" and "ah's"; and I was ready to throw in the towel when I suddenly heard an honest, clear, "Nice lines here," and then, "Lovely. Lovely." My father's smile, which had frozen—because he hated that we were both put on the line—thawed and his eyes twinkled.

When she came to *The Sprinter*, her smile became almost audible. To piece together any given moment I have to move my head very quickly in all directions. I mean, it's like several camera angles that added together make a movie scene or, better yet, like many pages of sequential drawings that flipped properly make a moving picture. I do it so quickly now that it's invisible— like the beating of a hummingbird's wings. But that day, between Marty's twinkle and Barbara's crinkle, and my own eagerness to see what she was looking at and each, individual reaction, I must have looked like I had Parkinson's disease as well as my own.

*The Sprinter* must be my most mysterious work. To me it is an athlete about to take off. To Henry Moore it was a mother and child. I don't know what Barbara thought, but laughing, she said, "This *is* suggestive, my dear." So there you have it.

I had my innings a moment later and I really heard the crowd roar.

"Oh, Gary. I like this very much. I can feel it. It must be wonderful to touch."

My father and I exchanged a happy glance.

"It's your favorite?" she asked, seeing the byplay.

"It's just that it's so great that you said that. It's titled *Touching Surface*. That's the name of it. *Touching Surface*."

"I think my foundry would be delighted to cast your work. Miss Moir will give you the particulars. They're good."

Quite typically, she later called the foundry herself to alert them.

"Do you have strong hands?" she asked me. "That's important. You must keep them limber and exercise them. I do, every day."

She then demonstrated fingers and wrists so double-jointed that I winced.

For three hours we talked and laughed, and then Jacquie brought in some booze—which I was still not drinking. My father, who fell in love with Hepworth, too, asked her permission to take some pictures of us. And then, every inch the English lady, she showed us her green thumb. I had never dreamed there could be a tropical garden on the Cornish coast, but that's what she had. Absolutely terrific; it was Eden. Lush foliage, great ferns, hibiscus and palms. It looked like paradise, and it felt like it to be there with this great lady.

Barbara now seemed to languish. I'm not a relaxing guest or a relaxing anything for that matter, and we'd been through a couple of lifetimes. Those three, intimate hours were the foundation of a beautiful friendship.

"We'll be off to France and Italy and then home and work. May I write to you? May I keep in touch?"

She touched my hand again and I felt I'd been knighted. This "difficult" lady gave me a book and inscribed it:

> For Gary
> With love and admiration
> Barbara

From my first love letter to our last brief conversation on the phone, just before a planned show of hers in Zurich a year later, we faithfully kept in touch. My work grew stronger. My health did not.

# 22

WE RETURNED FROM FRANCE and Italy, but not before I made my arrangements with Moore's enlarger, Henraux, saw the sights, selected some marble and ate the last of the puffed rice I'd brought to Europe. *Auf Wiedersehen; mein freund.*

I came home to Coconut Grove and never stopped working. I had five pieces exhibited at the Flagler Museum and, with Gene Massin's shrewd advice, I learned how really to price the many sculptures I was frantically turning out.

What a year that was. If, as the doctors had promised, it was to be my last, then it was going to be a winner. The three great sculptors of my time had encouraged me, even if the AMA had not.

I had been tough before meeting Barbara Hepworth. Now I was strong. I was stubborn before I met Barbara Hepworth. Now I was determined. Well, maybe stubborn, too. The chips were flying, the dust was settling. My father had lent me space in his factory now that I was into bigger work. Because of increasing transportation problems and medical needs, I sold my house and moved back to Palm Island with Marge and Marty.

In the middle of work on a cloud formation one day, I became dizzy, my mouth turned pasty and, aside from discomfort, I resented the intrusion on my work. Previously and periodically, I had put myself into the hospital out of boredom, caution and loneliness. Now I was too busy, but after seeing me Dr. Mintz asked that I have an IVP. A dye is injected into the veins in order to investigate renal function. It seemed that my kidneys, long victimized by diabetes and which had taken long-distance potshots at my eyes, were now themselves decaying. For the first time I feared utter immobility, dilapidation.

How was I to honor my promise to Barbara and myself if I was going to be the kind of sick that would keep me from functioning altogether? An organ here, OK! An organ there, OK! But everything?

With kidney failure, I began retaining fluid—bloating so that I was unrecognizable. My blood tests were worse than my math exams had been a few years before. Only the numbers were higher. This hospital stay was a bad one. I was given Lasix, a strong diuretic that made me lose the ten pounds I unbelievably gained in one day. Aside from my own organic gift for self-demolition, the dye that was used to diagnose me created a nephrotoxicity that, for a crucial period, collaborated in the kidneys' further destruction. I tell you, they get you coming and going!

I mean, I was really pissed off.

When I'd spoken with Barbara last, I had heard something in her voice, a vulnerability I hadn't sensed before. I knew that she herself was not in the pink, but she was as darling as ever.

"I want to be there for your show, Barbara," I said in a daze. "I miss you, but I'm in the hospital with a new wrinkle. I *do* want to be there with you."

"Then you will, Gary," she said.

*Yes*, I thought. *I mustn't forget that it's as simple as that.* "Then you will," became my credo.

I had the strongest feeling that Zurich would be her last show. I'd heard that she was fighting cancer and, strong as she was, she couldn't banish it as imperiously as she did other trespassers on her time and energy. Her voice was still vibrant. She sounded up and with it. I felt something though, and wondered if it wasn't simply my superstition or a response to my own mortality.

I needed to see her, be regenerated by her. I had gotten used to the lousy script I was enacting; and now, for the first time in about three years, Dr. Mintz was doing a rewrite. My melodrama was rapidly becoming stark tragedy. I wanted explanations and he gave them to me.

"What was this all about, Dr. Mintz? I mean, this last bit?"

"Your kidneys stopped functioning, Gary. They just stopped cold. They can't stop for long, of course—without preparing for alternatives."

"Alternatives? I'd hate that, I mean, really hate that—to be chained to a machine . . ."

I was sure he meant dialysis. He was talking transplant.

I couldn't absorb this new intelligence, but it precipitated a flurry of activity, starting with my signing papers relieving the hospital of any responsibility for the outcome of such a procedure were it to become urgent. I became acquainted with new, lovely expressions like kidney reserve, cadaver donors, tissue typing and the dreaded dialysis, which, as far as I'm concerned, robs you of all independence. It's a metal breast that makes you an infant utterly dependent on it.

I was in a whirl, the eye of the storm, calm and bewildered, uncharacteristically passive in the midst of all this dark and ominous action. Nature does numb you in the face of such news. It's called shock.

"A transplant," I heard myself repeat. "That's no problem. Just plug one in. You get them from dead people, right?"

"It's not that simple, Gary."

"Why not?"

"First of all, it's major surgery. Second, other people are involved."

"What other people? Who?"

"Well, we've found that most successful transplants are those from living related donors."

I tried to digest this.

"You don't mean—"

"The greatest success is with the immediate family."

"No way," I actually screamed.

"Gary—"

"No way."

"Gary, your family has felt so helpless up to now. This gives them the chance to do something, *really* do something."

"Oh, great. How generous of me."

"Look, Gary. We're not talking tomorrow, but knowing you, I had to share this information. There's nothing imminent. We've got plenty of time."

The whole business was unreal.

"I want to go to England, Dr. Mintz. I want to see a friend, an important friend."

"Maybe in a couple of weeks, if you feel well enough."

"I will."

*"Then you will,"* Barbara had said. But we hadn't known about a possible transplant.

My mother and father immediately offered themselves, each insisting that the other sacrifice the privilege of parting with a piece of his or her body. I couldn't believe it and flatly refused to accept either one. Weren't they afraid? Couldn't something go wrong? Parents or not, aren't their lives precious, too?

Dr. Mintz soon put a stop to that competition.

"Only blood and tissue tests can determine who will be the donor. Sometimes—"

"But I'm his mother!"

"I'm his father."

"Most of the time a sibling is the most compatible," Dr. Mintz interrupted.

"What?" my mother gasped.

"My God!" my father exclaimed.

"I will not have Glenn involved," I shouted. "He's only a kid and he's going around with Gise—and he's at college away from all this shit, at last."

Dr. Mintz raised the palm of his hand.

"I told you, there's plenty of time for all this. We're going to have to do lots of tests."

I just knew I had to see my brother. I flew to Northwestern. I

187

was to do that very often during his college career, but this trip at the end of his first year was unique. I missed Glenn and I guess I wanted to share this headline news with him. I could see his serious, slightly apologetic expression that veiled his intensity. He's such a subtle, classy, slightly loony character, my brother.

Always able to decode his message—from his earliest attempt at speech—I was, aside from noting a new remoteness, to be really surprised by him.

He had to know what was going on and there was no easy way of saying it. We sat at the edge of Lake Michigan, cross-legged on the grass. The day was brilliant and, as bizarre as our reunion was, that afternoon, the picture of it, was a quiet, lovely one. I was very low-keyed for me. And so both our voices were hushed as if the content of our conversation was too terrible to be heard.

Glenn was being quieter than usual and I inferred that he was still not adjusted to the big pond of Northwestern after having left high school a star. He had graduated with honors, was an admired athlete and winner of the Silver Knight senior award in journalism. Another winning Kleiman, but without the flak.

I was a tough act to follow, and he not only managed it but purified the family name. He had been a big man on campus. He was now a little boy in a strange place and, I gathered, also having an on-again, off-again time with Gise. On top of everything, I dumped my news.

Assuring him that I felt great and could handle anything that might come up, I also confessed that my recent setback had been more serious than I'd thought. Dr. Mintz had spoken for the first time of a transplant. Even now, as I write this, it seems unreal—an absolutely fantastic piece of information to convey to anybody. I spoke quickly, possibly trying to relegate it to the past.

"Are you ready for this? Mom and Dad are already fighting over who's going to give me the kidney. Typical. They're so great, but volunteers don't count in this fucking war. They may not have compatible tissues or something. We might have to turn to congenial cadavers—yeah, fresh corpses—how does that grab you? Ugh! He says that siblings can be the best donors."

188

I kept rushing on nervously, not being able to stop. What I was saying was out of a horror movie.

"So it's just conceivable, *not probable*, just *possible* that you may be nominated, but it depends on so many factors. I doubt if you'll be the hero but, well, you may be and I wanted to ask how you felt."

"Well," he said, his head resting on his fists, "if one of us has to, that's it."

Unlike his brother, he resigns himself to the inevitable.

This was the heaviest thing I've ever had to say to anybody. I haven't the foggiest how I, myself, would react if I were to be presented with such a contingency or duty or sacrifice or whatever the hell you call it. Because of my condition, I've always been on the receiving end of such devotion and generosity. Was he that punch-drunk from all the pounding? He just didn't seem to react.

"Anyway, that's the latest up-to-the-minute bulletin. They don't know when or where. I certainly hope to hell they know *how*. I guess you'll want to talk it over with Gise."

"Why with Gise? Why in hell with Gise?" he asked wildly.

And then I was really thrown. My horrendous disclosure, the possible threat to his future, wasn't anywhere near as awful as his wretched present. I now listened as the words came tumbling out of him. Life is so fantastic. There he was spilling his guts and needing me. I could still be big brother.

At this point, I had an army of doctors behind me, protecting my every flank and *achtung*ing all around the place. This latest campaign was sequential in the old battle for survival. But Glenn was alone. With nothing but his reputation for sainthood to comfort him. He was so damned self-reliant that everybody took him for granted, and here he was on his own and not doing so hot. It was the first crack in the armor that had both protected and stifled my brother.

The model student was lethargic and disinterested in his studies. He didn't care if he failed, was expelled or joined the foreign legion. Added to everything else, or contributing to everything else, my diabetes was as boring to him as it was to me. Now I'd heaped this garbage on him. The timing was all off. It was his turn to bitch. I needed him, or a part of him, just when he needed all of me.

Like, I mean, we sat on the edge of Lake Michigan that fine day and broke each other's hearts.

After a reportorial stint on the Miami *Herald*, Glenn gave our home a wide berth for a couple of years when he was on holiday. He became more and more distant and found jobs in New York and Washington, D.C., where he was miserable and worked as a copyboy for NBC.

When I visited him again in his junior year, he was unrecognizable. My formal, self-contained impeccable brother had now disappeared, and in his place was a zombie. He had transformed himself into somebody else. He had a wispy, scraggly, Amish beginning-under-the-chin beard that was *unbelievable* in its ugliness. Hippy remnants and John Dean glasses completed the picture. The chink in the armor had become a hole a mile wide.

Conversation was impossible. He had withdrawn to another planet. But underneath the disguise was Glenn. He was like a brilliant light bulb under a heavy shade. He'd had it and was sick of all the pressure to be a great student. He was sick of being a comfort to the family, sick of being the consolation prize, sick of being the calm after the storm. He wanted to make some waves himself. Why should I be the only one?

Glenn wanted to fail, fall from grace, be a villain and then be loved anyway. He hadn't really tested anybody's love yet. Shit, he'd been perfect. And perfectly sick of being the good brother.

He was doomed to be that forever. It had been scribbled someplace. His irrational guilt drove him farther into isolation and depression. Glenn really freaked out for a while, and I'm afraid I wasn't patient with what I thought then were elective troubles. I wasn't getting my necessary responses. Of course he wasn't either, but I'd unconsciously come to expect priority. This was like a bad day on the tennis court. We just weren't connecting. We kept missing each other's serves. And then there was that net between us.

My brother had always been Gibraltar in a Brooks Brothers jacket; I couldn't accept that he could crumble and come apart at the seams. There were two good influences in his life away from home. In addition to her feistiness, Gise had staying power and knew my brother's true value. For a tiny button of a girl, she has a giant and understanding heart. She should have gotten a purple one for sticking this one out.

Glenn's roommate at that time was going through his own growing pains. A very nice guy named Adlai E. Stevenson IV.

It all passed. Glenn made his waves and they carried him where he wanted to go. We became even closer with the years. It's now Glenn, Gise and Gary, the three G's. We even formed a 3Gs production company that produced a film for a class project at Northwestern. All for one, etcetera. Recently, discussing those years, we found it difficult to remember our precise feelings about each other. We evidently don't want to recall that time.

But it existed.

# 23

I T WAS MY MOTHER who got off the phone a few days later and
gently broke the news. Janet Chusmir had just called. She'd
just got the news from the Associated Press and wanted me to
know, wanted to offer her condolences.

Barbara Hepworth was dead. She had smoked incessantly. A
cigarette in bed. It wasn't the first time. It was surely the last.
There was a holocaust. They found her. It was smoke inhalation.

It was impossible to attend the funeral because it was so hurried and I was still under doctors' care, but I was determined to
go back to her house and her miraculous garden. My friend Mary
Ellen Taylor, the Thumper of my high school days, was then an
exchange student and was off to London on a summer session, so
we traveled together.

I called Jacquie Watson, who then told me that there had
been an inquest into Barbara's death. Though she had been losing her battle with illness, her death was determined to have been
an accident. She never would have destroyed her work or jeopar-
dized anyone else. There was going to be a memorial service in
London, to which I was invited, but, instead, Thumper and I followed Marty's route down to St. Ives, staying at the same charming inn.

Arriving after dark and retiring soon after dinner, we heard,
all night long, the terrible screeching of birds, the usually com-

plaining gulls now wailing—like albatross. It was nightmarish, and the natives said that they had never heard such an uproar before. Real bizarre. It was like nature was grieving.

In the morning we went over to the house, which was boarded up but still standing, seemingly untouched. I had imagined it would have been destroyed, but there it was. Stopping at her neighbor's across the way, I spoke with John Milne, who had worked with Barbara and who gave me what little news there was to give. She had been failing, suffering. At least that was over.

The sunlight was flooding the town—a Grecian light, she called it. The pretty village was at its best, everything in sharp relief; and I recalled what she had said. "We are all, forever, part of the landscape," and I felt her everywhere—in every landmark.

We drove down to Land's End, where I sat looking out over the water reflecting, writing some thoughts down. As terrible as her death was, I was glad that, instead of disease, one of her beloved elements had gotten her. I remembered the anguish she had experienced with immobility and "imprisonment" after her accident. I guess the shits had been after her for quite a while. Well, she had to be sleeping for them to catch her.

It seems astonishing that someone in whose presence I had only spent a few hours could have meant so much to me. But she did. Of course, our friendship was strengthened by many telephone conversations and letters, but her long-term effect on me was still, under the circumstances, remarkable. She managed to kindle my own sputtering sparks with her flame. It is odd that, in a sense, she consumed herself with it.

While I scribbled away at Land's End, I remembered that "on a clear day one can see the Isles of Scilly." Wanna bet? I stared over a grayish sea into nothingness and a startlingly white gull swooped down and perched very near to me, squeaking and muttering.

When I was very young, I thought that crying was a melting process, and if you really cried a lot, you'd disappear and become a puddle. I had raved and ranted for the last couple of years. I had bitched and sulked, but I had never really cried until that gray day when I sat there at Land's End.

My first major commission came soon after this—recommended by the seemingly ever-present Klines, who were instrumental in the first donation that involved us in the JDF. Sheila Kline called to say that Senator Gordon was building a bank in Hollywood and was interested in ideas for a sculpture to dominate its plaza.

After discussing my ideas with the senator, I built a model of cardboard and string and made a successful presentation, earning the commission.

Two stainless-steel forms that rise to a height of fourteen feet are joined by vertical and horizontal rods, all of which emerge from a pool. *Between the Lines* stands at the Washington Federal Savings and Loan bank in Hollywood, Florida, and it is a work I would, today, approach differently. I would simplify the forms, allowing their reflections in the water to complete the design and fill the visual space. It was still well received and I earned twelve thousand dollars for my first job.

Stainless steel is not cheap, however, and it cost me six thousand to construct. The profit was still considerable and I was so grateful to my doctors for saving what little I have of my sight that I used this fee to design and construct *Positive Negative Reflections* as a gift to the Bascom Palmer Eye Institute at the University of Miami Hospital in Miami.

This was a work I had first conceived back in 1974. I had gone to Gail Baldwin, the architect who had built our Palm Island house, and showed him preliminary sketches for a structure and fountain to dominate a plaza. One of my New York buyers, Michael Reilly, had paid handsome prices for my work and had recommended me to still another generous collector who was associated with the architectural firm of Skidmore, Owings and Merrill. He asked that I finish my designs and send them to him.

I thought Gail could help me, and I was really pissed off when he relegated me to his assistant, who was working away in a back

194

room—a kid my age and a graduate architect from North Carolina name of Sloan Marvin Burton III or something. I mean, come on. First Adlai IV, now this! Really out of my depth, I felt like I was *Jaws II.*

Bud was so pleasant and eager to help, and was so obviously a great guy, that I calmed down. We not only worked in vain for months on these renderings but became fast friends in the bargain. He certainly proved his friendship a few years ago in a New York hospital where I landed while he and I were on vacation and where—as I mentioned before—I felt so threatened.

I had developed a painful clot, possibly due to a medication I was taking for hypertension. After successful surgery, I was really out of it but still heard the nurses discussing my next insulin injection.

No matter my immediate problem—a common cold, a broken bone or indigestion—I am always diabetic; and so, while semiconscious and needing my shot of insulin, I heard myself warn them not to use Lente, a form of insulin that, especially under those circumstances, could have been disastrous. More concerned with this threat to their starched authority than with my limp body, they smiled condescendingly and continued to prepare this very injection. Bud and another great friend, Ilene Klein, came to the rescue and never left my side till my family converged on New York.

For Christ's sake. I did know what I was talking about. I've been forced to know. I tell you, keep out of their hands if you possibly can. First, you have to fight disease and then, when you least expect it, the people who've majored in it. When I'm conscious, which is most of the time, I keep my eye wide open for the menace of learned incompetency and graduate inflexibility.

This is why I wanted to show my gratitude to Dr. Norton and Dr. Blankenship, whose unquestioned ability is equaled by endless kindness, effort and patience. There's just no way of really thanking them; but I wrote the hospital that I thought the newly constructed building for the Eye Institute was great and I would love to donate a round sculpture to set off the square mass. It was

*195*

my "thank you" for their commitment. How awful it must be for gifted doctors to feel helpless and daily face patients seeking an impossible cure.

The hospital graciously accepted my design and *Positive Negative Reflections*, installed in 1976, stands proudly in that marvelous complex which is the University of Miami Hospital. I pass it every day as I go to and from the unit.

I now constructed *The Infinite* for the posh Quayside in Miami Shores. Alfred Browning Parker, the architect for the original project, had liked and bought an alabaster piece of mine called *Evolution*, a favorite that I hadn't really wanted to sell. It was he who recommended me to the developers. I love working with water, and the stainless steel was successfully delivered and set in a reflecting pool played upon by fountains.

Far more satisfying to me, however, is the fact that *Evolution* has found a home in this respected architect's office.

During this period, I was frequently called upon by the Foundation. Any time there was a need for a big push, a final plea for cash, they'd trot me out. I helped open a chapter of the JDF in Columbus, Ohio, and Cocoa Beach, Florida, near NASA.

My hyperactivity at this point was remarkable. I was on ten milligrams of Valium daily so I could sleep. I was making appearances, sculpting, writing lyrics and publishing slim volumes of poems and reflections that didn't demand public notice although the proceeds of my callow reflections went to the Foundation. It was my way of sorting things out. I was very young, sentimental, bursting to express my wonder, my love, my aloneness. Anything but my anger. The hard edge wasn't there yet. Just the hard times.

The country's Great Depression might have been in 1931. Mine was on our bicentennial, 1976. It started lightly enough and then went downhill all the way.

With all my irritations, it was difficult for me to cash checks without the only identification anyone in this land considers official—a driver's license. Mine had expired after the loss of my sight and my life was being made more difficult by this further inconvenience.

On my return from Chicago after visiting Glenn, I had the latest in arguments at the airport and decided, once I got back to Miami, that I would go to the license bureau and see if it would issue me a nonoperative license for identification only. As a sign of my growing maturity, I declined my city's invitation to mass murder.

"Wouldn't you like to take the exam, Mr. Kleiman?" the eager clerk asked. "You might as well while you're here."

I was complimented as always when people don't notice and I told him my problem, in detail.

"But why don't you try anyway?" he said.

"I don't think you understand."

"Oh, come on," was his only response.

Going along with the gag, I consented to look into some machine.

"Do you see anything?"

"No."

"Look closely." His voice was a trifle petulant.

I managed with great difficulty to read four letters. I was then given a written test which I held up to my lashes and painfully decoded.

"Now then," this born army induction-center doctor asked. "Have you any physical disabilities?"

"I have been trying to tell you for twenty minutes that I am legally, *more* than legally blind. I'm not allowed on the road."

This fellow became furious.

"If you don't want to drive, it's your business, but you've passed the test with flying colors."

I got my license—restricted for corrective glasses and a sideview mirror, the better to see what I killed after I killed it.

They obviously had concluded that my eyes were better than I and my doctors thought, because the law is rigid.

I really, legitimately this time, tripped over a chair on my way out.

If only I were able to drive, to go anywhere at will without being beholden. Can a healthy person understand what it is like to wait—always wait—for someone to pick you up and deliver you?

My chosen work in sculpture had isolated me, robbing me of that feedback I so needed from people, and now there was fear of even greater isolation and the dreaded immobility before and after the transplant. And there was now another terror. What if Glenn or my father (who would surely be the donor, we were so close) were to succumb to some surgical blunder or hidden vulnerability? Jesus. There was always a new load of shit.

Boredom has never been a problem for me. There hasn't been a dull moment. My problem is more like morbid curiosity. The question, "What's new?" is accompanied by clenched teeth by any friend who asks me.

For four years I'd been kept hanging. And not only about the chance of awakening any morning completely blind. Would I—despite impeccable care of my feet—suddenly discover an unhealing, festering sore that heralded an eventual loss of the leg? Would my bladder, my blood pressure or my heart momentarily send me into uremic poisoning, stroke or coronary thrombosis, all of these events on the agenda and not idle fancies? These were a few of the documented consequences of juvenile diabetes. There was nothing remarkable about me in this department.

And still, it was my nature and my will to ward off these eventualities, being more and more reluctant to accept their inevitability. My three-quarter blind faith in myself was such that I would somehow live with these possibilities. There was always the chance that I could keep beating those odds again and again. As with the unlikelihood of boredom, I seemed never to be cursed with the predictable. Since the complications, I had been on hold. Restless, it's true, but mobile. I was a *very* blue streak.

A transplant, I realized when I became fully aware of its implications, was going to change all of that. This was something else. I did my homework. People could *reject* the foreign organ, no matter *whose* it was, and that slight was not a forgivable rebuff, a social snub or a refusal to acknowledge, accept or appreciate someone's love. You *died*, pure and simple, unless you were attached to a dialysis machine, which for me would be worse. If your kidneys don't work and a replacement doesn't either, nobody's minding the store and it's *sayonara*!

I wasn't even sure, since a scratch was to be avoided, what surgery itself could do to me. And if I did survive the operation, would I then be forced into dialysis—often a lifesaver but notoriously dangerous for diabetics? My entire vascular system is so fragile now that the biggest artery of all—my heart—could give way.

And there it was. A whole new bunch of fears took hold of me even as I was conquering the old ones. Who was that guy who kept trying to push the stone up the mountain? He warn't no sculptor, like me, or he might have carved the stone, chiseled and modeled it to lighten the burden. Maybe I could make another Galatea, and she'd come to life and climb the goddamned mountain into the sunset—with me. It's worth a try.

What a year that was, 1976. Not one to celebrate alone with the rest of America. When I moved back home, I realized that I'd forgotten I took second place to the JDRF. The legend had really taken over the reality; the abstraction, the particular.

It was wild, unbelievable. The world was surely upside down and I dreamed of death. Of friends who had died, of Barbara, of a school buddy, of my grandfather, of an ancient white-haired man trudging through the Everglades searching, searching. Was it me? Was it *for* me?

It was three years since my hurried and ill-considered exit from Dr. Irwin Jacobs's psychiatric office ten minutes after arriving. I hadn't felt ready then. There was no question now. I not only needed help but *wanted* it. I couldn't have pulled my own tooth either, and this was all far more painful and deeply rooted.

As feeling as Dr. Jacobs was, he was detached—my first completely impartial ear. God knows I needed help. The first thing he did was help me face my rage. When I recognized how angry I was, I thought again of Glenn. We were angry for different reasons. I for being sick; my brother for being healthy.

It's really wild, sitting here, seeing the whole tidal wave instead of the ripples. The further away, the broader the vision. And even with the new panorama, nothing really changes. Things don't get any easier in this world. You just get better dealing with them.

Dr. Jacobs was the greatest.

"For Christ's sake, you'll burst—let it out. Tell me how unfair life has been to you 'cause it *has*. Get it out of your system. You're not a saint."

He knew me already.

"OK, you can't 'beat the shit out of diabetes,' then get a hammer and some nails. Shatter some marble. Beat the hell out of your beloved tennis ball. But get it out."

Once my anger was tangible, accepted as an entity, he was convinced that I could use it to my advantage. But first I had to release it. My poor mother. Everybody was to suffer, but Marge always got the worst of it. Gise used to call her "the battered Mom." It sounded like a headline in a tabloid. BATTERED MOM STRIKES BACK. But my mother never did. My slamming serves were not returned. She was far too busy trying to finance a cure.

It was exactly at this point that Janet Haas, my old tennis buddy, bumped into me. She was now pro at the Jockey Club.

"Gary! I haven't seen you at the club. Why aren't you playing? Any time you want to play a set."

"You've got to be kidding."

"Not at all. It isn't like you to give up tennis—or give up at all for that matter."

"Come on, Jan, this is a lot of crap. *I* didn't give up anything."

"Oh, I thought you did."

"Where have you been? Winning any cups?"

"I've been wondering when you're going to get off your butt and give it a whirl."

Well. I'm not exactly modest, and the idea of walking onto a court, especially one where I used to play tournaments, and falling over the net held little appeal to me. Being hit in the head by a serve was not my idea of a comeback.

"Forget it, Jan. Good try, get lost."

"I'll tell you what, Gar. If I can serve with my eyes closed, will you play?"

"OK."

She dragged me to my friend Jack Cooper's private court and she missed the first one. I howled.

"Never mind. Everybody gets two serves, right?"

"Right."

And then she nailed the damned ball.

"OK, OK. You've got a deal."

Janet now started punching balls to me like a teacher with a bloody beginner. It was awful. I didn't have any distance and I hit a few off the wood. I fanned completely and I couldn't hit backhand at all because the court disappeared. I mean, it vanished. I had to play open stance.

Then, after a while, I started picking some up and then I nailed a couple and it was real sweet. I thanked her for the fun and said that we would do it again some time. I then, for one whole year, secretly practiced against walls and then got my father to feed me balls at the net. We played like this as I prepared to take on Janet. Marty patiently stayed with it.

I gauged the distance, moving my head from left to right with those quick movements that couldn't be seen. I loved it and, anyway, a tennis court was home to me. My stamina was to diminish with the months and years and as fast as I was moving on or off the court, in honesty, I was getting progressively more tired.

I would jump around madly for a little while because I just *can't* do anything slowly; but then I'd fall apart and stagger to a bench and a Tab. But I was seeing the ball occasionally, sensing it even more often, being where I should have been more often than not. And I was playing, competing, able to be in control no matter how. Good or bad, with the ball landing in or out, it was always a clear-cut decision—and up to me. I heard the bounce and whizz and zing and I was making like I was healthy. I loved it. It was *really* twelve months, but I was ready.

"OK, Janet. I'm ready to take you on."

Janet didn't fool around. She's as competitive as I am, and although she obviously tailored her game, she didn't make it all that easy. That's not, thank God, her style.

When I was serving, I almost felt like myself again. A lot of the old force and some of the old direction were there. We volleyed around for a few weeks, and then one day, she insisted that we play a real set.

"Did I hear the word *impossible?*"

It wasn't all that bad. Because she's not a fraud, she won, 6–3. I mean the set was hers, but I did win a game or three. She allowed me to let the ball bounce a couple of times and I could play her double lines, but my pride kept me from permitting this. *There must be a way*, I thought, *to make it a more even game and still keep my dignity.*

Janet acted as if I were anybody she'd beaten. She'd fling her racket in the air or jump over the net and she never stopped challenging me. But I had to get even with her, so I devised my secret weapon.

I bought a pair of cheap glasses and black-taped one lens completely. I duplicated my own sight by taping three quarters of the left lens, leaving transparent only the bottom left corner. With the help of a pin, I added a point of light on the top right and then put cardboard blinders on the sides, so that no peripheral vision was possible. I brought the glasses to the court for our next game and handed them to her.

"Now we're evenly matched, girl. We will now compete in the Mixed Braille Open."

Janet was game, but I won it. Six to three. I don't know how she played at all. What a day that was. And what a friend this woman is. She helped me release a lot of energy and hostility, and it wasn't all that negative either. She really brought me back to tennis, which was my link to a healthier past. I've never given it up again, and am again playing every Saturday with my old school buddy Howie Orlin, the pro at Flamingo Park. It's great for me, but I think of those days long ago when I really gave Howie a run for his money. I was really good when I was a kid.

One day not too long ago—before the operation—I was playing doubles with three older guys who were only fair and didn't know me or my history. It was flattering but heartbreaking when one of them said, "If you stick with it, kid, someday you could become a real good player."

# 24

I F I EDIT all the garbage out of it, 1978 was a great year for me. I had my first one-man sculpture show, Landmarks and Steppingstones, at the American Foundation for the Arts in Miami.

There were eighteen fairly large pieces in marble, bronze and steel. An old friend did the catalog introduction:

> Sculpture is that link between the visible and invisible world. This awareness gives the work of Gary Kleiman its special poignancy. This is true of all of us. The world is ephemeral and what Gary does is what all artists do: catch a glimpse of the passage of visible into invisible.
>
> —*Isamu Noguchi*

I was really on the map now. The exhibition was a splendid success and I felt I had won at least one race. Let's face it. A venerable, white-haired old-man Kleiman with a sixty-year retrospective was not in the cards. My numbers were rising with my star.

The whole town, plus the crowd from the hospital and the JDRF, turned out for the opening. Dr. Meitus's daughter, Vicki, arrived with a group of classmates from Memphis State University. Fun, alive and responsive, they were really great. They were all taking a trip to San Francisco before returning to Memphis and school and I was eager to see them all again.

As the catalog revealed, I'd been working hard at my lonely

trade and I was ripe for people. Like a vampire bat thirsting for new blood, I flew up and descended upon them, meeting up there a girl who looked like Robin. She was studying to be a speech therapist and her father was an appellate judge in Tallahassee. I was impressed with Ginger Melvyn in every which way. She was bright, responsible and, of course, very pretty. She awakened those old romantic impulses that both attracted and paralyzed me.

Simple lust was easy for me. It demanded a fast approach that allowed for instant gratification. No problem. I'll die cocky. But *love*. That demanded distance and anticipation. At the very melting thought of *love*, an army of pious soldiers has always jumped to attention and taken its prescribed positions that would block my way to any successful campaign, no less conquest. I must revere, respect and worship—from a distance. Apparently I'm off the wall.

I obviously go insane when I sense the possibility of real involvement, and it may not be because I'm never sure why people like me. Being very sick is like being very rich.

All I know is that Ginger helped make 1978 a thrilling year; she recharged my batteries and turned out to be the perfect choice for my crazy adoration. She was forever to be in Memphis, Panama City or later in Chinook, Montana, where she worked with Indians. Talk about keeping someone at arm's length.

I needed therapy all right, and it wasn't for speech. Unable to declare myself properly with all my gift of gab, I could hardly have expected to elicit more than an echo from the young lady. I kept announcing that we'd always be *friends*, which was *forever*, and then wondered why we didn't become more.

I was forever saying lofty, bloodless things when I wanted so much more.

Dr. Jacobs has suggested that my romantic notions of women guard me against the distressing knowledge that even Juliet can have herpes. I don't know.

My relationship with Ginger was an intimate, long-distance phone call. Perhaps we were both playing it too safe. I was now so involved with my future, question mark, that my usual bullshit might have saved her a lot of heartache.

Though I courted her from afar, we did have fun when we were together, and loved sharing experiences. We laughed, we talked. I was programmed to save us from each other and she was obviously reluctant to break the computer.

Yes. With all my supposed and newfound enlightenment about myself, I was not going to burden this young woman. My halo should have been turned in for a dunce cap. She eventually became seriously involved with another guy. You will not believe this; it's unbelievable. He had—I swear—diabetes and *one eye*. I mean, what are they doing up there? Maybe there is a Weirdo after all.

At any rate, we have remained friends all this time, the result of many a stupidly handled romance. And we still share many interests. One of them is England. She has never been there and I am always lonesome for it. We decided that since we loved sharing so many things, why not a country? A solemn pact was made. If it was ever feasible to drop everything and go, one would call the other and simply say, "Now." I called Ginger last year and so announced myself.

We flew to London, the Lake District and down to St. Ives to pay respects to Barbara. England was wonderful, but I had taken Gary Kleiman along and I couldn't take my mind off an impending operation that might end, perhaps forever, all such spontaneous trips. I was moody, tense and altogether shitty in my unreasonable demands for perfection in the universe. I just couldn't understand why nobody else seemed to try as hard as I did to make the impossible a reality.

Going back to the end of the seventies, I was asked to enter a Dade County competition for an art project meant to enhance a day-care center in an underprivileged area of Miami. The Department of Housing and Urban Development had allotted one percent of its appropriation to art. That meant, in this case, that there was about a thirty-thousand-dollar commission.

I was certainly gratified when I won and delighted as the concrete *Playforms* became an eight-foot-high and twenty-foot-long reality. Without Barry Massin, Gene's son, an industrial artist, I'd have been lost. For ten years he's been my right arm and both eyes. If I have any question about basing or engineering a piece—and I always do—I run straight to him. More than once, I've been called an executive sculptor.

With *Playforms*, we made a Plexiglas model from my design (derived from hundreds of sketches) and then it was permanently cast in concrete. It was designed to be climbed up and down on, crawled in and out of and certainly scrawled over. The kids loved it and it was a great honor to create a setting for laughter and sport. I felt it was sort of Hepworthy. I think she'd have been pleased. But when I went to Tenth Street one day to photograph the structure and rap with the neighborhood people, their response was not very warming. The police protectively suggested that I leave. I didn't feel very privileged. It was really sad.

It was then that I was recommended to do a large piece for the Miami International Airport. I didn't have too much hope, because it didn't seem apt that I be the city's sole sculptor, but nonetheless I designed *Wings*, one of my favorite works. The architectural committee loved it, the Art Council loved it—only the nonvoting members loved it. I smarted for a while and was reminded of Bernini's statue in Rome's Piazza Navona that for all time points its mocking finger at St. Peter's dome, the commission for which went to another.

I was more than consoled when real estator Martin Margulies, who was then building Grove Island, a complex of hotels and condominiums in Miami, selected one of my stainless-steel pieces for his International Garden, which graces the whole island and accommodates one of the finest private collections of sculpture in the country. I am exhibited in the finest company and still cannot believe that I stand out there in the sun, casting my own shadow along with those of Moore, Nevelson, Smith, Calder and Noguchi. Incredible. I have no complaints in this department. I'm a lucky son of a bitch.

I had met Marty Margulies through the Foundation's Nancy Marumsrud, who was seeing him before her marriage to Martin Kahn, the last president of the Foundation. The gentleman had been to my exhibit, liked the work and made the mistake of saying he might consider one of my pieces for his project. He had only one building of the magnificent project completed, but suggested that I keep in touch. He hadn't quite meant for me to call every day, but I did. I was ridiculous, relentless. I knew about his collection of modern painters and sculptors and his plans for an immense outdoor sculptural garden. I had staked a claim on a piece of that virgin acreage. His phone never stopped.

"I am sick of your calling," he informed me when next we met.

"I'm sick of your *not* calling," I answered, trying to be funny.

"What?"

Martin Margulies was a youngish man but hard of hearing.

"I'm sick of your *not* calling," I repeated.

"You're a pest."

"Yep."

"You're really persistent, aren't you?"

"Yep."

"OK. I'm going to give you a break. I'm sick of getting your messages. Will you stop if I buy a piece?"

"Yep. I promise."

"So do I."

We both kept our word.

I believe that Marty owns more Noguchis than anyone else in the world, along with his single Kleiman. We greeted Noguchi, the one and only, one night at the airport and all dined together later at Marty's. I was waiting to be picked up and expecting a call.

Isamu was so funny. He was disappointed in the Bayfront Park design and ill at ease at the overwhelming Hotel Kenilworth, where Marty had put him up.

"My instinct is to flee," he whispered. "I'm rattling around here. I'm out of scale."

"Your phone, Marty," I interrupted, hearing the ring. *Are all Martys deaf?*

"What?"

"Your phone."

"Oh, thanks. You tell me when it's ringing and I'll tell you where it is."

Noguchi couldn't believe our routine and took refuge in thoughts of another project.

If one artist can really teach another, Noguchi's lesson is clear: Choose your medium carefully, know exactly what you want to accomplish and then work as hard as you can to do as little as possible.

I guess I took him too literally. Satisfying as my success was, work had become a chore for me and removed me from the great, big wonderful world that at any moment was going to be unavailable.

The suspense was unbearable. Dr. Mintz hadn't been kidding. I discovered that my body had to be very sick before a transplant could be successful and save my life. I had to be much sicker, but my eroding kidneys were taking their toll on my strength. I still had the usual reactions to diabetes, but now I was really always fighting fatigue. The autointoxication resulting from my body's inability to wash away its impurities was draining me of everything else. Frequent visits to Dr. Mintz and my own medical kit kept me abreast of the lousy news. My creatinine count was up there. All of it terribly elevated but holding. "Normal" readings are usually less than and no more than one.

"When you get over six, we'll have to start moving. You have time," Dr. Mintz explained.

But how much time did I have? All my friends, everybody around, were making plans—either to get married or take jobs or sign up for postgraduate studies. It was ridiculous for me to make plans. What kind of plans? Where to have dinner? Who was I trying to kid? Would I see the outcome of the national election? Would I make what now seemed the inevitable wedding of Glenn and Gise?

While I still had enough strength, I took a three-and-a-half-week trip to Europe with my very literary friend Mitchell Kaplan, and it was the greatest holiday I'd ever had. I don't think I could have spent that much time exclusively with anyone else. An old friend from school whose parents were friendly with mine, Mitchell is not only a really brainy character but a remarkably accepting one. His understanding of my clinical needs and toleration of my sometimes insufferable life-protecting self-indulgences were remarkable. How he survived my hypersonality and I his patience, I don't know.

We traveled through England and Norway. I probably will never again enjoy such freedom and spontaneity. Those quaint old days of simply taking insulin, examining my blood sugar and contemplating my goddamned pee were over. My present daily regimen sounds like a four-year course in medicine.

Of course, not many others would have made the trip in my condition to begin with, but I was raring to go and, Jesus, I love to move, to go, to run, to see, to live!

We hit London, went to Devon and, of course, Cornwall, then north to Windermere and Edinburgh and on to Newcastle, where we took a boat to Bergen, Norway. We stayed in a converted dorm in a youth hostel and that was where I got sick. I couldn't stop urinating; it was like I sprang a leak or something. I lost so much weight that most of my strength was gone. This diuresis panicked me, so I put in a collect call to my nephrologist, Dr. Goldsmith, who never panics. Carl Goldsmith, luckily, was brought into my life by Dr. Mintz at the time of my renal shutdown. Without question, his brilliant manipulation of drugs helped delay the inevitable transplant by seven years. He's one more member of the great team I've been fortunate enough to have.

"Drink a lot, Gar," Carl said. "It's just dehydration. It's nothing terrible and it's no surprise."

It is true that before I became the world's leading authority on diabetes, I was kept in the dark by my doctors. They withheld information about pending symptoms because they didn't want me to anticipate nature and suffer them prematurely. I understand that now; but, without warning, I was never sure—when something like this would arise—that the incident wasn't terminal.

With all my complaints about the great, healthy past of mine, the trip was a breeze except for that moment. I was safe with Mitchell. He knew my whole, boring saga and all the pitfalls of bumming around the Continent with a diabetic. The frequent stops for food, rest or medication. The possible incidence of reaction, and even hospitalization, which necessitated my lugging along an international list of doctors. Mitchell was prepared for any- and everything and rolled with all the punches.

There were so many inconveniences—with my salt-free diet, especially in Scandinavian restaurants, and my goddamned eyes, which had me talking to strangers instead of Mitch who had stopped at a bookstore a minute before. Nothing diminished my excitement and joy in acting like any old healthy tourist. We ad-libbed everything. No Eurailpass, no accommodations, no idea where we'd land next. I loved it. We proceeded on whim and enjoyed every moment without reservation.

Replenished with plenty of orange squashes and Perrier, I was reconstituted and able to continue our tour. I really did feel like instant coffee or something. "Just add water—"

We took an express boat to Flåm and then down to Oslo through the Sandefjord inlet, which must be the most beautiful sight on earth—besides a creatinine reading of one. We sailed through towering, icy cliffs on a ribbon of gorgeous, blue water, so deep that it had sheltered English submarines during World War II. The mountains were conversely as high, astonishingly lofty and narrowing the sky as waterfalls spilled and sprayed silvery water. Everything sparkled in the sharp, dry air and we truly lost our breaths. It was Cinerama, yet fellow travelers—evidently commuters and workers—were changing toy boats, going off to tiny towns, kissing each other's cheeks and taking all this grandeur for granted. What a spectacle and how wonderful that I could see it.

Mitch and I went on down to Copenhagen and then to Amsterdam, and if I had my way, I'd spend the rest of my life in flight. I should have been a bird. When someday they examine me at leisure, I'm sure they're going to find vestigial wings.

# 25

**M**ITCH AND I have just flown back from another New
York weekend, doing the galleries in search of a Moore
litho I thought I'd get my mother. I also saw Glenn and
Gise and caught up on some theater. I had a tough week with the
kids last week and needed the change. This morning, back at
work at the unit, I saw one of my more difficult patients.

Fourteen-year-old ungainly Sally and her slim beautiful
mother do not address each other at all. The wall between them
was obviously built as a joint effort. Sally is lethargic, shrugging
away the chores that, undone, are taking their terrible toll. Her
waistline and bad skin shout of contraband sundaes and pastry.
You sort of wonder, observing her listlessness, how she manages
to negotiate it all. While her mother recklessly speaks of blindness and amputations in a vain effort to get a rise out of her, Sally
sits dreaming of revenge and feasting on desserts that could, by
sending her into coma, end her terrible existence. It is astonishing
how self-destructive she is; and yet, it is understandable, I guess.
For behind her glazed expression, there is a hint of triumph as she
thwarts her mother.

This is an act of, a fantasy of, revenge. Her gluttony and indifference to her own needs will be the punishment that fits the
crime her mother committed by being, first, beautiful; second,
"giving" her diabetes and third, never getting off her back
about it.

It is far beyond right or wrong—if actually I could know which is which. Ironically, I must be an ally to both. If I say her mother is right in wanting her to be strict, I will only be joining forces with her greatest enemy and send her into more stubborn resistance. The poor mother, however, is on a righteous rampage and has forgotten, really, what the crusade is for. No matter her sincerity, if the only thing she is going to accomplish is the reverse of what she wishes, then why? On the other hand, she can hardly do nothing. But I must get Sally to work for herself.

"Sally, I know it's unfair that you can't eat what you want—and *when* you want. I know it's lousy."

There is no reaction. She just keeps biting her lip since nothing else is handy; and she stares above my head at the wall.

"Who in her right mind wouldn't want a banana split instead of two Lorna Doones?" I persist.

"But she could go into coma and eventually—"

My nod of acknowledgment stops her. Returning to the girl, I say, "Sally, I bet you're as upset as your mother."

She shrugs her shoulders but nods slightly. There is a glimmer of recognition behind her sullenness. But still, can the kid trust me? At least now there's a possibility. I never mention her fat. She knows she's fat and hates herself for it already. Her mind is working in a different direction. Is she pretty? Could she possibly be prettier, so that the "boyfriend" whom she always quotes to rile her mother will cease being fictional?

After seeing her records, we make changes in her medication, but despite my work, the time together has not ended in any victory. This is a slow business, gaining her trust, returning any self-esteem she may once have had while still not alienating her mother. If the woman is too intimidated, she will remove the child. So it's the devil and the deep. I just know, for sure, that Sally must feel that I understand her rage and frustration. I'll learn more next Tuesday. Without her trust, my counseling is worthless. And without my counseling, my life would be another story.

\* \* \*

It was about five years ago when Denise Skyler, the diabetic nurse specialist at the Children's Cardiac Hospital, called me. Her husband, Dr. Jay S. Skyler, who's all brains and energy, heads the diabetes unit at the hospital and has since become my boss there.

For two weeks a year, he also runs the Eagle's Nest Camp near Asheville, North Carolina. It is part of the North Carolina Camp for Children with Diabetes (NCCD) and affiliated with Duke University and the ADA North Carolina chapter. As a matter of fact, I'd first met Jay Skyler at the Rice House and then often ran across him on my many visits to the University of Miami Hospital. Because of the Foundation and my local show-biz notoriety, Denise asked if I would help her with a patient.

"We don't seem to be able to reach him at all. He just won't cooperate. I thought because of your sports, your accomplishments—the kid has seen you on TV—you might be able to get to him."

It was always clear that I got on with kids. At my youngest and most wicked, I was always careful about kids. Ever since I'd first seen Glenn, pressed his belly button and got his private messages, I always had loved kids.

It was also true that I was finding it hard to grow up myself, that I understood kids and they felt at ease with me. Add to this my credentials as a bona fide, dyed-in-the-wool veteran diabetic and it became increasingly apparent that I was about, at last, to find my true vocation.

Denise's problem boy was my first patient. To the Skylers and the rest of the staff, he was another recalcitrant. The woods were full of them. But to me, as Marc and I faced each other in Dennie's office—the desk our "net"—both of us taking the other's measure, I found I was face-to-face with myself. It was chilling.

In this thirteen-year-old boy, I saw the depression, distrust and rage that was eating me up between accomplishments and laughs. Marc's mere presence in a hospital was an affront to him. He belonged on a playing field. Complications hadn't touched him yet, so denial was still possible. I stung with the recognition. I could match him play for play.

Marc was rebelling against parental authority. Fifteen all. He was crazy about sports, hated restrictions and didn't want to be set apart from his teammates. Thirty all. I don't think he liked himself. That was never a problem with me. Forty-thirty. My serve. Marc was only thirteen and could possibly still mend his ways in time. Deuce. Marc was convincing himself that, if he ignored his illness, it would go away. He wasn't taking his insulin, which is like playing Russian roulette. I was a bit too self-protective for that. My advantage.

His depression was global, all-inclusive. He wouldn't apply himself to his studies or his health, a contrived civility replacing genuine human exchange. Myself at Duke, except that I didn't even pretend to be civil. Marc is sweeter. He bowed, as I did, ever so slightly to the authority of the doctors, but mumbled monosyllables for answers. He wouldn't address the problem with any logic. And why the hell should he? What the fuck is logical about diabetes?

Marc had become an emotional hermit pretending ignorance.

Except for my days at Duke's Rice House, I hadn't been near anyone diabetic except in the countless reception areas and corridors waiting interminably for my doctors. For years I had been the diabetic boy in a healthy society raising both money and hell when I could. I caught his long, hard look of appraisal. What new, boring speech was he going to get now?

I really, honestly can't say that I devised a means of reaching Marc. That first meeting was an extraordinary one for me. Now, of course, I'm an old pro. I know all the tricks and have learned much from Jay and Dennie; Wendy Citrin, diabetes psychiatric social worker, and Debbie Seigler, physician's assistant, with whom I work so closely at the unit. But, then, the first time I didn't have to be experienced. It just came.

"It's really shit, Marc, isn't it? I mean to have to give so much fucking time to this garbage?"

He hadn't expected this. Perhaps I didn't either. I just knew what he was feeling.

216

"You look fine," I continued. "You usually feel OK, except for *those times*, and who needs all that work—for what?"

Marc was silent.

"Isn't that true? It's a drag—the records, the blood, the piss, the numbers. Right?"

"It ain't fun."

"No. It ain't fun. That's for sure. I used to hate it, too. I once drank my insulin when I was a kid so I wouldn't have to use the needle. Jerk!"

"No kidding. For real?"

"For real. I swear. I got *real* sick. I still hate it all—the whole bunch of crap—I always will. You'd have to be out of your mind to *like* it. I mean, come on, man."

The kid grimaced his assent and almost smiled.

"You know why I always do it, though? Why I never miss a day? Because for me, *personally*, I like being in charge. I don't like letting anyone else take over."

Marc looked away thoughtfully.

"That's just me, of course. I don't like people telling me what to do. And let's face it, I don't like feeling shitty. Jesus, I've felt sick even when I've done my best, so I'd have to be a real nerd to bring it on on purpose. You know what I mean? I like myself. I didn't always," I added quickly. "Wetting my bed and getting sick and stuff like that was a big drag. I learned, though, that I could take charge, and now I love my work, my tennis—"

I wondered if I should go on. "I was pretty dumb as a kid and, well, I didn't take care of myself."

"You look OK to me."

"Yeah! And I am. I keep myself pretty busy."

"So?"

I was on dangerous ground giving such an impression of health.

"I thought you were the guy with the eyes?" he continued.

"Quite a description. Is that how the police would find me in a crowd?"

"You know what I mean."

"Yeah, I know what you mean."

I took off my glasses.

"I get by just fine, as you can see." This was my first attempt at juggling. "You'd never know, but I just may not have had this fucking problem if I'd taken better care of myself when I was your age."

There was silence again.

"This doesn't happen to everybody, Marc. It's luck, I suppose. But, you know, I wish I could go back and take charge earlier, when I still had something to say about my own future. I don't want to trust to *luck*. It's tough though. I know it is, Marc."

"But I feel better when my sugar is high so—"

I knew he was both denying and giving himself reason to indulge himself. But there's something else as well.

"Are you afraid, Marc, of what happens when the sugar gets too low? Are you afraid of reaction?"

I remembered myself in that London hotel.

"I hate that feeling," the kid answered.

"Tell me, Marc. Are high sugars good for you?"

"Well—"

"Well, are they?"

"No. No, I know they're not."

As Dr. Mintz once said, "Kids have the answers. You just have to ask the right questions."

Marc was sitting stiffly, uncomfortably, waiting to be released, waiting to be out in the street where no one would know he had diabetes and he could "pass." He was stiff and unpliable. If I couldn't mold him, I'd try whittling.

Maybe it was selfish and I really wanted to be in charge of more than myself. Maybe with all that identification I felt, I saw for the first time the probability for a second chance. Whatever, however, I got to him. I couldn't cure the kid and I couldn't make him carefree, but, damnit, he came to know that, flawed or not, he is a miniature of that architectural marvel—man, unique in nature because he can make decisions that are not only reactive but creative. Marc came to know his own worth; he called me a few days ago to say he was off to college. So far, so very good.

After my meeting with Marc, Jay and Dennie asked if I would see more kids, at least once a week. My work as a volunteer grew to three days a week and I always felt wonderful after being with the children. Wendy then had me sit in on classes for patients and trained me in techniques. She and Debbie Seigler are both great with kids, and—aside from their knowledge, high spirits and dedication—just kooky enough to reach their charges, who in turn adore them. Since I'm not the sanest man in the world, we make a triumverate—the unholy three—who troubleshoot, interchange our patients and remain, even when out to dinner or on dates, available.

I would have to be dying or dead before I'd call anyone at 4 A.M., but these kids do it all the time. Just last night. They call any time the spirit moves them, since self-absorption seems to be one of the symptoms of this disease. They call if they're sick, if they can't sleep, if their parents are giving them a hard time or if their parents are too permissive.

Never dreaming that I could be so gratified, I looked forward to those days with the kids. Of course, I was still sculpting, but not selling a lot. Dennie suggested that I fly up to Chicago and see her grandmother, a rich old lady who collected art. She owned Giacometti, Arp, Hepworth—name them. She lived on Lake Shore Drive and like many old people, she had lost the knack of whispering. She bought nothing and when she introduced me to a man from Christie's, she put her gloved hand over her mouth and shouted, "His eyes. Give the poor kid a chance."

I flew home to Miami and asked Jay Skyler if I could work at the unit full time—for pay. I will always be grateful to him.

As my complications multiplied, my attention span uncharacteristically became more undivided. I've mentioned "feedback" a couple of times and how important it's always been to me. My patients and my new friends gave me this in spades. It is my fifth year at the hospital. The kids and I need each other and that makes me the luckiest bloke around.

Dr. Mintz conducts, among other things, a sophomore course on the mechanics of disease at the University of Miami Medical

School, and every year, at his invitation, I join him as case presentation and emotional stripteaser. The students ask pertinent questions and I answer them impertinently. My case history is fascinating to everybody except me. It certainly can be instructive, I suppose.

In this course, Dr. Mintz wants to convey to his students the impact of disease on the individual beyond its symptoms. He wants these future doctors to address themselves to all the issues that rise out of and subsequently pervade the entire life of the patient and his family.

Year after year the students will ask the same questions. "How much information should be shared with the patient?" "Do you tell him about the possibility of severe complications?" "Do you thereby, in a sense, contribute to them, or doesn't it make any difference?" Smart lads. "Frankly, Dr. Mintz," another adds, "I, too, am a diabetic, and as a med student this is a double-edged sword. At times I'm afraid to hear things and, then, other times I want to know everything so I can adjust to the worst and deal with it. I don't want to get like that. [He was pointing at me.] I think if that happened without preparation, it would even be more damaging than anything."

"Like that!" The kid was certainly going to have to develop a little tact. What a bedside manner!

It's a difficult question to answer. I personally want to know everything. I don't like surprises. And even as I say this, I know that I hear too much in the elevators and commissaries of the hospital. Candid as he has always been with me, Daniel Mintz, because he is wise, knows that there is no certainty in anything— even man's fallibility. He therefore always holds out hope.

This same kid now said that, when his girl friend came to visit for the weekend, he was startled when his blood sugar went sky high. He wasn't aware that he was under the pressure he usually felt, for instance, before an exam, and therefore had made no insulin or caloric adjustment.

There is that eternal vigil, evaluation and juggling act that can be upset by an intangible. Like most of us, he was trying—for

220

the next time—to gauge himself through precedent and reason. Ha! I relieved his present tension somewhat when, observing his priority of stress, I asked him how his girl friend's blood sugar was. Well, you know!

Another student, after hearing how every patient's tolerance of grim reality must first be determined by the doctor before information is shared, raised his hand, stood up and shouted, "But this is sentimental. This is the twentieth century and Gary was just saying how important it's been to him to protect himself from ignorance and pie-in-the-sky optimism that might have killed him and caused his retinopathy. I believe the patient mustn't be spared anything. I don't believe in beating around the bush. He's gotta be told the worst right away—right on—so that he can prepare himself properly, even for death."

Dr. Daniel H. Mintz, the biggest softy around, stared at the student who'd run out of steam and had sat down.

"You will please take your notes and your things and leave this classroom, which is for future doctors," he said. "You don't belong here."

Even I was surprised by his coldness and vehemence. The student turned white and actually trembled. He seemed about to respond and Dr. Mintz repeated, "Please leave this classroom."

The entire class sat in embarrassed silence as the guy gathered his things and slowly made his way to the exit. It was a terrible thing to see. As he opened the door, Dr. Mintz stopped him.

"Come back to your seat, young man. Now you know what it's like to have—in one split second—your whole future taken away from you."

Dr. Mintz knows how strongly I feel that techniques and procedures formerly reserved for physicians but which are now commonly available are *required* information for patients. It is true that "they are the real managers of this disease on a minute-to-minute basis all their lives."

And he agrees, in my case particularly, because he knows me. I am both his patient and his assistant. He wants to share, when possible, as much data as possible, because he really believes that "the metabolic effects of diabetes can be controllable, and microvascular complications can be prevented and ameliorated."

We sure would like to think so, and frankly, I'll settle for a stalemate, a tie. I put all my energy into the fight and hope only that nothing else negative will occur. With control and intelligence, the possibility is lessened; without them, there's just that dumb luck I talked about with Marc. I think I would go stark raving if I had to relinquish my life to chance.

I mean, who says you can't change things? We're changing the face of the earth, why can't we change the heavens as well? Maybe some new people will move in up there.

When I was a boy, my parents asked me if I wanted to go to a camp for diabetic children and I, of course, refused to go. I was sure I'd be branded forever, be considered a freak. I played at being healthy and went off, instead, to a regular camp where I so neglected myself that on that one brainless, foodless, all-day canoeing trip, I had the terrible DKA experience and was sent by ambulance to a hospital.

Like Sally, Marc, Robert, Rinaldo and hundreds of my other kids, I had to learn the hard way—by growing up. Some of us with diabetes have not been so privileged. I've been fooling them now for ten years.

When Jay and Dennie Skyler asked if I would like to be a counselor for two weeks at their camp in North Carolina, I jumped at the chance. I was curious and, most importantly, I could move my ass and be in the midst of the action.

222

# 26

Eagle's Nest Camp is in the Pisgah Forest near Asheville, North Carolina, actually nearer Brevard in the Blue Ridge Mountains. It's really nice.

I wasn't really prepared for a two-week love-in. I mean, it was—with all the hard work—a fourteen-day high. There was so much laughter and music—and caring. These kids have learned, despite what Wendy calls the camp's collective grief, just how precious life is. Early on is the time.

A lot of people find the camp sad. I can understand that, although I see the other, crazy, healthy side. It is true that the sight of five-year-olds with their own medical kits isn't exactly happy making. They're all graduate doctors by the time they're six or seven. Or so it seems. Little mad scientists with vials of blood and urine along with charts and colored crayons. With everybody taking shots and all the accompanying music, it's a Lilliputian version of Woodstock.

Gise and I were talking about it the other day. It's incredible. Instead of feeling like freaks, all the kids from five to fifteen do their chores not furtively but openly. Because everybody's doing it. It must be the way Jews say they feel when they go to Israel. The cop on the beat is Jewish, the banker, the telephone man, the manicurist, the hard hat. They're not singled out or *think* they are being singled out. They belong to the majority at last. The same with the blacks in Zimbabwe.

But as in any group of people with a common ritual and a genetic fraternity, the individual must be developed. A great supporting cast may be important to the kids, but families and camps, supporting casts, can disappear and the patient may be left on his own. He must find himself resourceful.

One of the great milestones in my life was my realization that, despite my extraordinary family, doctors and friends, I depend mostly on me: for firsthand information, unequaled familiarity with the case and undying, uninterrupted devotion to the cause. My will for survival is so great that I must trust my judgment, if not all my motivations, more than anyone else's. Of course, I don't know if I'll survive my parents, doctors and friends, but I must prepare myself even for that contingency. Imagine that gall, considering my prognosis and my often-voiced belief that there are times when I swear I only go on for them.

It just goes to show you.

Whenever Marge slips and says something like, "When I'm seventy and you're fifty," there is a noticeable moment of silence ended by my, "And what about when I'm ninety and you're one hundred and ten in the shade?" Every individual handles this situation differently, and I have my MO.

Eagle's Nest Camp is a group like any other in so much as it is made up of individuals. It is made homogeneous only by a common disease. Ten to fifteen young individuals are in each cabin, along with a clinician and a counselor who are in charge. The clinician is usually a third-year medical student or physician's assistant from Duke, the University of Miami or the University of North Carolina. The clinician obviously is medically responsible for supervising the management of the camper's diabetes while the counselor, usually without medical credentials, is the camper's adviser and friend, in charge of the overall well-being of the cabin unit. As the camp calls it, gestalt. He or she must help the camper adjust to group living and, just as necessarily, his chronic illness.

For the very young children, the camp is a kind of diabetes kindergarten, providing these first lessons in their continuing education and lifelong defense against the disease. They are instructed in proper diet—a subject of highest priority. They learn, at each meal, to balance the prescribed forty to fifty grams of carbohydrates with the necessary protein and fats. They learn to make preferred exchanges—like fifteen french fries equal two slices of bread—and they come to understand the need to adjust their rations of food to their physical activity.

If they are going off for a long hike or an exhausting game of baseball, they can increase their intake of carbohydrates and even take the opportunity to indulge a little, knowing that the sugar in the cake or Coca-Cola will be burned off quickly. They come to know that they must avoid sweets as a natural enemy and also devour them as an antidote in case of hypoglycemia. Food to a diabetic person is both an indulgence and a medication.

The children, in order to make their regimen easier, must try to eat uniform meals every day so that the dose of necessary insulin needn't be that hard to reevaluate. Even with this, a common cold or emotional upset, even a dream in the night, can demand a dramatic readjustment. Therefore, the essential dextrometer, or finger-pricking blood test. They must, at every moment, be aware of the need to balance food, insulin and activity so that their blood sugar will never go too high or low.

And then, as they grow older, they must learn the difference between the types of insulin, which, incidentally, are much purer and more effective than they were when I was a child. There is the regular fast-acting insulin, the intermediary Lente, NPH and the long-acting Ultralente or PZI, which works for over twenty-four hours. Then there is the combination of these that must, with more mature consideration, overlap but be carefully calculated. Back in New York when I was lying on my butt, the Lente that was prescribed by those idiots would have eventually thrown me into a real episode, because it would not have taken effect when I needed it but would have exceeded my sedentary needs once it did. The eventual refinements of knowledge are astonishing, the curriculum endless, no matter to what degree you aspire.

If the preceding has bored or overwhelmed you, just imagine the kids!

The moment the camper unpacks his bag and receives his

own mini-medical kit, before the raising of the flag and the grace before breakfast, he or she learns that

1. Diabetes mellitus is a permanent disorder, a lifelong condition that is possible to control and impossible to cure.

2. Self-care (and he will be instructed in those disciplines) is essential and will be routine—like eating and sleeping.

3. The patient is not alone and can have professional help at any moment.

4. The camper will, with only a few restrictions, be able, in fact encouraged, to do about anything a person without diabetes can do.

At camp, at home or abroad, every boy or girl with diabetes must be knowledgeable about the disease. The moment afflicted children are old enough they should be able to

1. Define what diabetes is.

2. Understand the primary factors controlling blood sugar, that is, insulin and exercise.

3. Be aware of the effects of physical and emotional stresses on blood sugar.

4. Recognize and treat hypoglycemia.

5. Evaluate and adjust his/her management and control.

6. Detect impending and dreaded ketoacidosis, coma, and appropriately intervene.

7. Recognize the implications of continuing glycosuria, or abnormal amounts of sugar in the urine, and their significance in terms of future complications.

8. Realize fully the importance of general hygiene and health, specifically foot care.

I set down this long but partial list to remind the reader that these are children who must acquaint themselves with such necessary bullshit. These are children who must, every single day, conduct themselves with the discipline and dedication of adults in order that they may someday become them. If I belabor the point somewhat, it is because, to this day, I am astonished by the amount of time I spend just staying alive. I'm used to it. It's a challenge and I've got it licked. But I'm dismayed, to say the least, when I see these kids already groaning under the weight of what is a lifelong burden.

It starts when they open their eyes in the morning. The boys can have their first void in a Dixie cup—in bed. The girls have to drag themselves out of and back to bed. All the beige, plastic kits are now opened. They hold cubes of sugar (in case), washable test tubes, droplet pills and dropper, insulin and needles. The kids can test their blood sugar on a glucometer and pray that they will read a count of 80 to 120. They also cross their eyes in hope that their urine is blue, not orange or brown. There is tension every morning, suspense every night.

Is it any wonder that my mother and father still shake with anger when they remember being comforted by the sanguine doctors when I first got sick?

"Thank God," they gushed, "it's only diabetes."

I've had to take a year or two off from camp. The operation has made that necessary. These are not just diabetic patients, they're kids, and like all new things the bugs haven't been removed yet. The joint is swarming with germs and I'm not exactly in the position to ward them off right now, or probably ever again. There's always the chance, especially with the younger campers, that there'll be a little measles, mumps or chicken pox or just a freckled, running nose. For five years I always came home with something, most of the staff did. No. I'll have to be wary of working at Eagle's Nest again, and that's one of my highest mortgage payments. They were happy days for me.

"Thank God, it's just diabetes." Something that will stick to you through thick and thin, stay forever at your side. Loyal to the end. And having said that, it is, nevertheless, my daily commitment to convince the very young that they must make do. At both the unit and at camp, our first aim is to encourage a positive attitude and an acceptance of diabetes. It's a reality, like a Siamese twin, and you must live with it with grace and good-natured vigilance. The technique is tough, but it can be learned and passed on to others. It's like spinning a lot of plates aloft on tall

227

sticks. The more you practice, the easier it gets. If you keep at it, most of the china remains serviceable.

Every single day that I make the act work, I seem to be able to get another booking. Practice makes the imperfect bearable. I really don't mean to sound like an idiot, but nothing is impossible, and your grasp has to exceed your reach. You do this alone as an individual; but places like Eagle's Nest Camp can aim you in the right direction and help, through training, to supply you with the unnatural stamina necessary for success.

At places like Eagle's Nest, some of the kids get the proper dosage of insulin for the first time. I was horrified to discover that, in many communities, insulin is only prescribed once a day. Towns far removed from big cities or universities are especially remiss. I can only guess where I'd be today if— Jesus! Imagine being stuck in Magnoliaville with bronchitis and having cups put on your back.

Destructive patterns are changed at camp. And the children, along with their parents, are taught to demand the right treatment. To someone who had suffered alone though surrounded by love and care, I saw the remarkable modification of unhappiness in such convivial company.

Peer pressure and approval were factors that had never occurred to me. Cruel as they can be, children can and do encourage each other in real crisis. The overheard conversations that follow are accurately recorded. Believe me.

"Have you tested your piss yet, Jim?"

"How many units are *you* on this week?"

"You really handled that last reaction real neat."

"Gee, do you want to get dizzy and fall asleep? Where did you find that lollipop?"

"Come on, Anibale. I'll help you with your shot. We're going to be late for breakfast. Come on. It doesn't hurt if you do it right, and you gotta *know.*"

"I'm afraid."

"Here. I'll do it with you—together. I mean, at exactly the same time, and then I'll race you to the hall."

228

These are the campers. All in the same boat and, because of that, less likely to sink. I wonder what I'd be like if I'd had that kind of interrelationship as a kid. The awareness. They really feel responsible for each other.

But these are still children and we, at camp, must never forget it. In case of nocturnal emergency, honey is kept in each cabin. It disappears sometimes. As seriously as they approach their illness at one moment, they will then fake illness for a reward of sugar cubes, too young to know about "just desserts." Their precocity is not wisdom. What a conniving, manipulative, dissembling bunch of wonderful brats they are. It could be a reformatory where the punishment fits no crime unless it be original sin.

Wendy is the greatest of "guards." She is appalled by what she sees in the camp, but she never communicates this and never descends to destructive sentimentality. Like everyone who works with children, sick or healthy, she doesn't always feel adequately wise to handle a special moment. This lack of confidence we have all felt is, if revealed, epidemic. As she puts it, "Intangibles enter the picture and you're completely thrown. How can we be absolutely sure at every given moment that we're right? Well, it isn't necessary to be right—just effective. If we help, it's right."

She manages to ask questions whose answers make any judgment of hers unnecessary. She never seems to punish or diminish these already victimized boys and girls. And still, in her catechism there is discipline. Watching her in action is something. She seems to convey her disapproval of a child's behavior even as she empathizes with it. And the kids get the message. Bingo! Wanting her approval, they try to mend their ways. Wendy taught me that the child should earn his or her *own* approval. And I'm the guy who can second that.

I've learned plenty from Wendy and Debbie, who also operates with a velvet scalpel. Debbie's good. When she's giving me transfusions, she never worries the veins but teases me. She's always been one of my links to the OR, operating room, to anyone who's never seen *The Doctors*. Debbie is real hospital-wise and has prepared me for what could have been many surprises. When

I get real fresh, she tells me to go jump; she's a real close friend. She's another tough one, but she can't hide the tears always ready to well up. She's emotional like Gise. It's hard to believe she manages to go from patient to patient, feeling as deeply as she does; but like the rest of us, she's developed a technique.

While I was waiting for my transplant—and she and Wendy and my family were waiting along with me—one of her patients was a guy who had had a transplant after a double kidney and spleen removal. During dialysis, this guy lost his vision totally, and Debbie was spending time with him, not knowing what to say or do and, of course, saying and doing all the right things, because she cares.

When the poor guy complained about a meal plan or something and said that he had this restriction and that restriction and he wasn't goddamned well going to have another one, Debbie sweetly said, "Sorry, Charlie. You can argue all you want. I'm not arguing back. Have you forgotten why we're having this little chat, how we happened to meet?"

All of this in her crazy southern drawl, and he got it. She was having those feelings of inadequacy and guilt and was also shattered by his condition. But she was effective, because he dialed in on her.

"I guess you've gotta be a drill sergeant sometimes," he said quietly, perhaps feeling her own need for help. They both felt better.

I tell you, these women, along with another friend on the hospital staff, Adrienne Keller, are great to work with. Being both counselor and patient gives me a different kind of clout, but I've learned that when I have a problem with a kid, I never structure a scene of reproval and pose at my desk while a child sits defensively on the wrong side of it waiting for punishment or, at the very least, disapproval. I always work my spiel into a natural conversation or, at the camp, always got my licks in on the way to the lake or playing field. The off-the-record, spontaneous response to a breach of rules or personal crisis seems to work best. I can make a good pitch but, you know, kind of curved—with a little English.

As eager as we are to build confidence and self-reliance, if a kid stubbornly insists that he wants no parental or staff interference, that as a smart nine-year-old he's capable of independence, I simply agree. I suggest that he move to New York or San Francisco and get his own apartment. Bingo. The kid invariably laughs as he flounders. I still don't use my advantage. I simply concede that his rights must be respected, like everybody's, including those who love and care for him—and even some people who have diplomas for learning how to help him.

The group dynamics achieved at camp taught me plenty that first year. Trusting the kids doesn't automatically make them trustworthy, and my better eye has always stayed open to disobedience and sheer devilry. Remember, I wrote the book on those two. But you try. And then there's a whole relearning process through socialization techniques. The corrective factors of group psychotherapy are impressive.

"You mean you don't get angry when people ask, 'Can you eat that?' "

The need for catharsis or self-pity—just one cc, though.

"I don't blame you for bitching. That's really the pits."

The recognition that others have the same problem and are struggling, too.

"I'm not the only one like this."

"Your way seems to work better than mine—I think I'll try it."

The resultant unconscious altruism.

"Maybe I won't be so depressed if I can help *you* a little."

That one's a real beauty.

And love.

One of the diabetic junior counselors, whose younger brother was recently so diagnosed, confided that as rebellious as she's always been, she had never once felt guilt. Not until now.

"I've been a terrible example for him. Terrible. But now *that's going to change.*"

Incredible, how dedicated she became. She wouldn't do it for herself, though. We must encourage patients to think and appraise themselves. The question I always ask is, "What do you really like best about yourself?" It really starts the wheels going.

I was already committed to working with these kids at the unit, but my own transformation, I think, was completed one day when I had the children on a picnic.

The countryside was a brilliant green, the breeze summer sweet and the river eager to host all the brown, wriggling, squealing bodies that were now braving the rapids. It was all laughter and vitality. These children were just like any others, and then in the midst of all this vigorous, spontaneous play, it was suddenly time for insulin shots and the forest primeval turned into a kind of obscene M*A*S*H.

On another occasion—a long hike—one fine day following a rain, our group was happily exhausted and starved for lunch after the arduous walk. Because we had hamburgers and spuds ready for cooking and we had, as always, planned the exact insulin, exercise and diet interactions, there had been no need for supplements on the long trek. A perfect day could have turned into catastrophe, however, when the still-wet leaves and twigs smoked but wouldn't catch fire and lunch had to be perilously delayed. There's not much margin for error with diabetes.

I have just got back from a two-day visit with all my old young friends. I decided I could go for a couple of days if I was really careful. Our diabetes unit purchases spots for thirty to fifty children every summer and, this year, since I was unable to be there on duty, I managed, through some promotion and good friends like Dr. Jacobs and Marty Margulies, to angel the plane fare to and from the camp for the entire staff and the thirty-eight kids involved.

Of course, the Foundation responds quickly to our requests, as do the Miami Springs Junior Women's Club and the Pan American Clipper Club, whose generous members are the pilots' wives.

Since my kids and I correspond and the campers and I missed each other, it seemed wise—as well as selfish—for me to visit, if only for a day. I missed Eagle's Nest. It was important that the kids know I was OK.

I play a dual role all over the place. First, I am proof positive that you can beat the odds and, second, a grisly assurance that neglect can only earn debilitation. No boxer has to be as fast on his feet.

This year Gise, a second-language teacher of children with learning disabilities, asked—because of me and because there's nothing that doesn't interest her—if she could visit and volunteer at camp as a counselor. After she arrived, Wendy took her under her wing and then let her loose. What a natural. Gise was marvelous after she got over her initial shock. As is true of most people, she couldn't take seeing so many sick kids in such an incongruous environment. The first evening, she saw a boy, fourteen, carry an unconscious nine-year-old back from the playing field up the hill to the infirmary "like a GI lugging a wounded buddy behind the lines." The matter-of-factness of his manner and the generally mild interest from everyone else drove home what she felt was the apparent familiarity of the scene. Fortunately, that extreme is rare.

It threw Gise, who's quick to tears. She survived the initiation and the tears dried, leaving the salty Gise I know and love. She takes no crap from anyone, including the kids.

Since she is authentic, the kids loved her. She hasn't a phony bone in her perfect, little body and her eyes narrow in the presence of phoniness. Gise was there for the whole two weeks and fit right into the picture. She not only learned fast and was a great counselor, but the kids went ape.

Attention-getting little Cathie—a born actress—who has parlayed her diabetes into a long-running soap opera, ran into the cabin one day, the back of her little hand against her forehead. With suitable pauses, she declaimed, "Gise, Gise, I'm having a *reaction!*" and started swooning. Our Gise took all the necessary precautions but sweetly said, "Honey, I would call this an *over-reaction.*" It was obviously Cathie's first notice and led her to develop her style as well as a crush. She was to learn some restraint, in everything.

233

Children, of course, really love grown-ups who won't take their bullshit. As long as they feel real interest, they crave authority. Gise was to see more clearly than most the terrible harm so many of the permissive parents did these, her temporary charges. "It's wild," Gise told me in New York on her return north last week, "the Latins are all Jewish mothers. They worship their kids and won't even let them take their own shots. They do *everything* but void for them."

Unfortunately, despite the fact that after two weeks at camp the boys and girls become more self-reliant, these new disciplines are sometimes almost immediately destroyed by parents who descend on the camp the last day, sweep their children up in their arms, slobber over them and renew the preexisting dependence. The two weeks go down the drain if the control returned to the kids is usurped again. It would be wonderful if there were a camp for the whole family.

It is the diabetic child himself or herself who needs to know and thoroughly understand the short-term effects of excesses—immediate sickness—and the long-term results of laxness—complications. The kids actually have asked us to intervene and urge their mothers and fathers to allow them more self-discipline. But this sovereignty is not to be interpreted as license. We know the kids who want this. Their own will could atrophy if not exercised. I have even on occasion come across a child who is too meticulous, really compulsive in his need for self-ministration. This is a different problem, one to be handled by doctors. I know we have to make a career out of our illness, but there are workaholics.

There's no end to the variations. Shockingly enough, some of the parents happily dump their sick son or daughter in the camp and then resentfully or fearfully have to retrieve them. Some actually resent their sick children and have themselves, for years, denied the illness until it has become so unmanageable it has to be faced. It's then that they find it a pain in the ass.

With the less-informed parent, the imperfect child reflects some hidden sin and all the unwanted guilt that goes along with it. The child becomes a buck passed back and forth between the

234

parents, each denying responsibility and recalling some remote relative "with sugar" on the other side of the family. There is also shame. But mostly these parents find the whole business a nuisance and damned expensive, both of which it is.

This terrible state of affairs usually remains out of our hands, and we can deal only with the negative effects and suggest guidance. The kids are burdened enough without the additional weight of all this crap.

The boys have possible impotency to fear along with everything else in the future, although corrective measures can solve this problem; and the girls have another bonus concern. In her cabin Gise was exposed to the fears that have been voiced to me back at the hospital. Twelve-year-olds brooding about the dangers of eventual pregnancy. Not on behavioral, but purely medical grounds. Can they give their husbands children? Healthy children? And will they themselves survive?

Today, with care, drugs and diet perfected, diabetic women, under impeccable control, have a good chance of normal birth and recovery. One of my patients in Miami, Cindy Hooper, was so grateful for any help I might have been through her pregnancy and labor that she honored me by making her undiabetic baby my namesake. The poor kid's name is Gary Hooper. Cindy had fears, as most female patients have, for the baby more than herself, and we all relaxed when she had a textbook delivery. But this fear of pregnancy and childbirth starts early.

"I don't think I should ever become a mother!" thirteen-year-old Veronica confided to Gise one evening after my sister-in-law had given the smallest kids their shots and tried to clean up what she properly considered a filthy cabin.

"I'd be afraid, and it isn't a good idea," the child continued. "I don't think I could handle it."

Gise was tired.

"Nonsense. You'll do just fine, Veronica." She then fell onto her bed exhausted. "Just don't have fifteen kids with diabetes living in one cabin with you."

But then Gise would whisper to me, "Look what they all have

235

to do in order to play like kids; I mean, they're babies." And her eyes moistened again.

"It's good for them, Gise. Believe me. They work to play, but they might as well know the price for everything right now, so they won't be too stingy to pay it later. Nothin' for nothin', man."

One morning when Gise brought me some milk to take with my Cyclosporin, I was doing my thing. The whole production. The glucometer, the insulin, the pressure, the Cyclosporin, and I suddenly became aware that Gise was watching me. I turned and caught her amazement. Throwing my arms in the air, I leaped a couple of feet like Nureyev and then bowed deeply. Gise gave me a standing ovation.

"Every single day, Gar? I mean, a few times a day?"

"And twice that on Sundays. Then there's the early-bird performance."

"You really accept this," she marveled.

"Very reluctantly, Gise. I don't accept it any more than these kids do, but I deal with it. There's no choice."

Gise's eyes started filling up again.

"For Christ's sake, Gise. Cut it out. This is me, the old con man. I can handle it. This is the least of it. I've got a grip on things."

But her eyes were getting redder and the tears were now falling.

"Gise! What is this shit? Stop crying."

"I'm not *crying* and I'm not worrying about you."

"No?"

"No. There's something wrong with my damned eyes."

Par for the course!

Like everybody else who ever was enriched by a visit to Eagle's Nest Camp, my sister-in-law came away with more than she'd bargained for. She returned to Connecticut with conjunctivitis.

Far more lasting as a memory is a conversation she overheard between two of the older campers.

"Would you tell your girl friend about your diabetes, Freddie?" asked one hesitant boy obviously mulling over the pros and cons.

"Of course not."

"But supposing you had a reaction while kissing her?"

"I'd just swipe the bubble gum out of her mouth."

Freddie is another one who will make it. A real natural selector. And that's what the whole damned shebang is all about. If your lungs go, then try breathing through your ass. If that fails, try something else, but don't give up till they carry you off screaming.

# 27

CREATING BEAUTY or a new way of looking at earth and its teeming life—art, if you will—is great. The desire, even the compulsion to share your vision and change the future is what makes our species special. I learned to model shapes out of chaos at the clay feet of masters. To temper steel and cleave marble, to carve wood and cast bronze is miraculous. To alter space felicitously is God-like. I'm busy on a basic design for a new commission now, and I'm a happy if undriven sculptor.

It was only when I started working with young people that everything really fell into place. My father had told me that my most important job was staying alive. It was apparent that diabetes, one way or another, would be my career, but I didn't know that it could make me happy and encompass so many people.

One might say that my work was cut out for me and my business expanded. With my commissions, my hospital work, my good friends and loving colleagues, plus my own private driver, Nancy Politis, who materializes like a pretty genie whenever I need her to take me hither and yon, wherever they are, I had it made, except for the ever-darkening sky above Miami Beach. I was fighting it, hiding it, but feeling lousier by the day, and I didn't have to be clairvoyant to know that what was left of my kidneys was goofing off.

"You mean I have to be even sicker than this?" I asked Dr. Mintz.

"You've got to be even sicker."

It didn't seem possible. My creatinine was now over five and a half. A series of tests was being conducted, and there was lots of shadowy action behind the scenes—conferences that suggested possible surgery in Boston instead of Miami. Boston was one of the five centers to prescribe the use of Cyclosporin, the immuno-suppressant that Florida had not yet sanctioned. Of course, surgery was still just talk. I didn't believe it was going to happen anyway and just went along with the gag.

Through my Aunt Tobia, who is a volunteer worker for the New York Association of the Blind's Lighthouse, I heard about a projected commission that fascinated me. It held the possibility of creating a sculpture in some way related to blindness.

My professional involvement in the lives of hundreds of troubled young people had somehow made my sculpture seem a frivolous self-indulgence, and art itself somehow hollow and nonfunctioning. Mere aesthetics, unrelated to humanity (which, of course, it never really is) had ceased to interest me. I felt an urgency to say and contribute something more to the world around me.

But The Lighthouse changed all of that. Here was a chance to combine my two interests. Obsessed with time, I sketched some designs for bronze pieces that I hoped would make tactile the twelve months of the year. The cold, the heat, the patterns of rain or snow, the textures of the sand with the receding sea, barren-ness, foliage. It was fun to do, and I sent slides to my aunt, who forwarded them to one Wesley Sprague, who kept them after showing some interest and then apparently forgot me.

In order to construct any of these designs, however, I needed funding, so I applied to the National Foundation on the Arts and the Humanities. I didn't fit into the proper or specific category or something and that too seemed kaput.

With my creatinine stabilized at about five, nothing seemed to be resolvable. And then I was saved by the bell.

Mr. Sprague called. I flew to New York, saw him and Mrs. Donald Stralem of The Lighthouse and learned that a sculpture was needed for the brand-new Pisart Award funded in her will by

239

one Mme. Georgette Pisart, the widow of a Belgian diplomat. For many years she had been a volunteer and supporter of the institution and now had bequeathed an annual, tax-free fifteen thousand dollars and the still-to-be-designed award to that man or woman who "during such year shall have distinguished himself or herself by invention or otherwise in prevention, cure, treatment or care of blindness."

The next thing I knew I had the commission. Since the award was to be given to that person who would have, in his or her achievement, somehow altered light and, in a sense, redirected vision, I now had a job that took my mind off of numbers and dates. I wanted my design to be organic and not some figurative, sexless form that poor Oscar has been cursed with. I wanted something abstract but also optical. A prism within a globe encased in a crystal sphere was my first idea, but it didn't describe the puzzle that is blindness. I didn't visualize anything trendy. It had to be classic, since the award was in perpetuity or at least long range. Although most of the audience and probably the winner would be sighted, I wanted it also to be aesthetically pleasant to the touch of the blind.

Because the award had to do with vision, and vision with rods and cones that are responsible for light and color perception, my unhappy familiarity with such matters could be used positively. I had fun mulling it over in my mind. The prism and the triangle had always knocked me out. A four-cornered structure can be wobbly; the pyramids have been with us forever. Such strong and beautiful forms. As for the prism, its shattering and rechanneling of light, its bending rainbow, its mystery fascinated me. I had studied Buckminster Fuller's geodesic dome, made entirely of triangles.

Aside from all other problems, it was necessary that there also be a logo; this meant that my design would have to look good in two as well as three dimensions. I did six models before I was satisfied. Finally, using three sections of a vertical rod, each cut at forty-five-degree angles and standing at different heights, I was able to achieve the upward, regal motion that I sought; in addition, when seen from above, the puzzlelike shape—which is the logo—was revealed through the hollow prism core.

All this sounds like I'm just Mr. Wonderful, but, after my initial conception with cardboard, I went to my pal Barry Massin—always my first step. "I need a rod of clear acrylic and at the flattened top I want to draw an equally sided triangle and then extend the lines from each point to the circle surrounding it."

We cut the rod on a band saw, and then I removed the prism, creating the negative. The conception was executed. It worked and we loved it. Accepted by the board at The Lighthouse, it was magnificently fabricated in crystal by Orrefors in conjunction with Tiffany, which did the sterling base. This entire project and everyone involved in it were perfect, right down the line, but I wasn't sure that I would be able to make it to the first presentation. At that point I didn't know whether I would make it to the next Dolphins game at the Orange Bowl.

"Dr. Mintz," I begged. "If the Dolphins make it to the Super Bowl and I go over six and you've got to operate, could we do it at halftime?"

It may be that the whole voyage of my life has been an ego trip. I don't know. I do wish I were purer in my motives. I love being in charge with the kids and their bewildered parents. I love wearing that beeper on my hip and playing at being Marcus Welby or somebody. Action brings corruption and I'm hyperactive.

From my first TV appearance, I discovered that discussing my descent into heaven actually took my mind off my trouble. The medium blurred the message. I'm certain that there have been times when my family has suffered more than I have. I've been spared nothing except the sweep of the drama. *They* have had to watch me.

I didn't understand this until the whole family was being type-matched and had blood and tissue tests. Glenn, when we got home that day, looked at me in wonder, and then alone together in my room he broke down. I had never seen him that way. "How can you take this? It isn't fair. It isn't fair." His grief, so terrible to witness, came to enrage me. Such raw suffering shattered and burdened me with more guilt to carry along with all the other shit. I felt so helpless that I almost freaked out. I mean, I lie a lot of the time to my family about how great things are, and that's shit, too, but it's easier to handle than consoling them.

Gise told me to get it off my chest, and Glenn and I had a real heart-to-heart and it was better.

When I was expected to have the operation in March 1981, Glenn called. "So this is it, huh?"

"Yeah."

"I'm not *quite* ready for it."

"Neither am I."

"Yeah. So don't do it without letting me know, OK?"

It's really tougher on them because they—all of them—can't know. There's just no way to *know*. They can wonder and imagine and feel for me, but I'm the one who knows. It took a long while for me to relinquish my monopoly on suffering. Why shouldn't other people suffer honestly, openly? I had redesigned, framed and advertised my pain, displaying it my own way. My lamentations had been published as reflections and corrupted with meter. Watching a loved one in anguish is a terrible thing.

Was this what I had done to the whole family these ten years? But this is why I kidded around, why I was so outrageous, why I laughed so quickly. If I laughed at my disabilities, I trivialized them. But, of course, they knew that. They're smart. Where the hell had I been?

Glenn and Gise couldn't afford, for Christ's sake, to donate twenty-five hundred dollars to the Foundation. But they did. They were just married and needed every penny. What was this guilt? I could have brained the schmuck. I *want* him to have the world by the balls. I love it that he brought Gise into the family, that he's got the woman he loves. It's one of the bright spots in my life that he's so *with* it. I knew when we first met that he'd be OK; I loved him when he had nothing to donate but a wheeze and a dirty diaper. I *don't*, however, want to see him suffer because of me. That goes for my mother and father and anybody else. I've got enough on my mind.

I know that I'm selfish in my demand that others not reveal their reflected grief. I'm a shit. But the guilts start to pile up, each resonating from the other and growing in a kind of mathematical progression. I guess I'm impossible, but so is my life. I don't have time for all that garbage.

Poor Glenn. He's watched my dwindling life quietly, in that dreamy, gentle way of his, and only broke to me that once and only because he, rather than I, recognized the enormity of the pending surgery.

With all that jazz I'd always heard from doctors in the past, I also, more recently, had heard the serious music. Jesus, I work in a hospital—with diabetic patients. Too many things could go wrong. Anything could happen. And what about my eye? There was a tremendous risk of losing my remaining vision by waiting a moment too long.

"I know you want a date, Gary, a time. I can't say exactly as yet. When the damage is irreversible, we'll operate. It will be *very* soon."

I had, at last, found myself and had gained strength through revelation as much as pigheadedness. I had survived ten years by thumbing my nose at the fortune-tellers and fighting. And now I'd been told that my body had to give up in order to survive. What a dilemma. To make things thoroughly pleasant, my blind eye had started to give me severe pain. Talk about insult to injury. It may eventually have to be removed, the glaucoma pressure is so great. Well, live for today is my motto, and have direction tomorrow, just in case it comes.

My work continued at the hospital and the studio. I was talking to Dr. Jacobs about writing this book. I was dredging up memories and taping conversations with my friends. There was an idea for a piece, a commission. There were several ways to approach it and I had to decide fairly quickly. And, I kept playing tennis, though I don't know how. Badly I suppose. Finally, my

243

numbers were getting higher—five and a half again—and we were put on the alert.

The donor kidney was at last chosen and the drumroll started in the distance. From someone already hyper I went into double time. I wasn't going to miss a thing.

"What would you do if you were told you might only have a month to live?"

It must have been the parlor game at the Marquis de Sade's. All the guests fill their glasses gaily and then delve into their psyches.

"I'd take a trip around the world."

"I'd rob a bank and buy the most gorgeous chick for sale."

"I'd tell my boss to go fuck himself."

"I'd tell my husband to go fuck himself."

"I'd kidnap Brooke Shields."

That's the parlor game. It's not the way it works in real life. Real people cry their eyes out, OD or retire to their God.

Me? I refused to consider the possibility.

# 28

I F ONLY I COULD blink my way back into Barbara's garden. It was so quiet there, and beautiful. I'm back at Jackson Memorial Hospital, where they're giving me a triple renal scan to determine why everything isn't working perfectly. It seems that every time my sugar count goes down, my creatinine goes up. I'm doing all right, really, but we aim for perfect.

Dr. Mintz, in answer to my incessant questioning, has implied that even with success, there is always the possibility of further surgery. I'd kind of like to keep what I've got now, even if it's sometimes wanting. You do get attached to the parts of your sum. I don't want a plastic eye, either. It may be a poor thing and painful, but it's mine, all mine. Lying here, there's so much to think about. There was this woman recently—before Judie—who said, "I never met a man like you before," and I really got hung up on the word *man*. She called me a man. I can't believe I'm not a little boy anymore; it's weird. It really threw me.

"You've got to be sicker."

The depleted body obviously stops fighting the invader. That's what makes the chances better.

How do you know when you're close to death? I mean, so close that the next inch does the trick? I've never felt that way. The tennis just gets lousier along with my mood. We wait and wait and wait.

No one knew how I was walking around, much less working at the clinic, playing tennis and keeping up the social life that has always nurtured me. I was literally at the end of my rope. The last sliver of hemp was about to give way. Like a movie when the mountain-climbing hero's line has been worn away by a jagged rock. In a moment—hold your breath—it could snap, and then the inevitable fall from frame with only the slowly diminishing, echoing cry of *"Help!"* filling the void. Real dramatic.

As always, I removed myself from this reality and watched the perilous scene from a loge seat. It has always been my way of handling horror—the stepping aside and becoming the fascinated spectator. *How will it all end? Will the rope hold until a helicopter or friendly eagle repaying some former kindness saves him?*

A rush of panic, a thrill of terror may seize me momentarily and then that marvelous suspension of belief, the detachment and the necessary polishing of my image. *Brave, funny and quixotic Gary Kleiman is indomitable and always triumphs and returns for the next exciting chapter.* Between you and me, it's a hell of a strain. The performance is continuous, but it's not a one-man show. The whole gang is part of the cast, all of them acting their hearts out. My family, my friends. Everybody bright and sassy, picking up their cues before they're even thrown.

At work, crazy, wonderful Debbie and Wendy, who know better, being pros, were now discussing the impending surgery with all the lighthearted optimism and wild banter they usually reserved for romances with the wrong guys. Only Dr. Jacobs asked right on if I thought of the transplant operation as a life-or-death proposition and I realized that, insanely, I really didn't. I thought of it simply as being restricting. I felt, quite rightly, that my leash was going to be shortened, that I would be out of control for a long while, that my freedom rather than my life was being threatened. My conversations with Dr. Jacobs couldn't have been more honest, but they had the same sense of unreality. I was sensibly discussing someone else's problem. I was caring and somehow uninvolved. I tell you, it's great to have an immortality complex, especially in the light of all this shit.

Years ago, I decided that my life would not, despite events, be a tragedy. My family and all those I love were not going to be subjected to that, and there's too much fun around to belabor the horror. I'm not feigning indifference to the threatening implications of my condition. It's only that I refuse to accept them as immutable. Underlying my sickness there is a very healthy guy trying to overcome and bust out.

I guess I set the tone early and resolved that if I couldn't realistically win the big one, I'd at least fight the bastards to a draw. They might even get worn down and, like Marty Margulies, say, "If the bugger wants it so frigging badly, what the hell, let's give him a break."

Horrible as it may be, diabetes has been my closest companion for a quarter of a century. There's something almost touching about its constancy in this ever-so-changing world. I marvel at its fidelity, its sense of purpose. I know its ways.

The reality of the projected transplant was a different story. All the predictables went out the window. This was a new situation, perhaps as inevitable as my other involved complications, but this was revolution. I had lived with the eventuality for years, half believing it would never be necessary, trusting that my will would keep my creatinine to a level that wasn't "sick enough" to demand such a giant step.

Yes. Diabetes was a treacherous buddy, but we had developed a kind of detente and I had learned how to conduct myself. Now that the operation was just down the corridor, I had to make some rapid readjustments. The silver knight had to shine up the armor, reshoe the caparisoned horse and get back on the tightrope. I'm not mixing any old metaphors. I'm trying to give you a picture of the situation. Slightly improbable.

If I dropped my guard and lost the edge of control, I could, by stepping on a tack or a sharp shell on the beach, bring on gangrene and, in its wake, amputation. What then could major surgery do? Could I even survive it and—if I did—knowing my

247

stubborn streak, would I resist and refuse to be host to the new kidney? The timing of the operation had to be exquisite. I'd been twinkle toes for years, prancing along between the devil and the deep, and this much stayed the same. If I was relatively too healthy, my body would fight off the new organ which, after all, was a foreigner and, to the brain and its many minions, an enemy to be attacked. How the hell could I explain that this was one immigrant I'd lift the quota for, one invader I would welcome?

Then there were other complications. My hypertension was a prime concern. Could the trauma of surgery bring on a stroke? Of horrifying import, would the previously mentioned immunosuppressant Cyclosporin, which would with luck as well as calculation permit me to accept this exotic savior, be so permissive that it would, with no discrimination, now allow a hundred killers free access? We know there's a price for everything. But the cost of living has really gone sky high.

Surgery remained imminent, but we were all ready for it. For eighteen months. And reexaminations of myself and the donor were necessarily brought up to date in case of organic changes. The suspense was almost insupportable, but you go on. Since life should be a continuous process of evolution, I must say that, under fire, my character was tempered. I started out wild and willful, and that hasn't changed, except now I'm wild and willful about the right things. I've boiled my emotions down to those relationships and activities that matter. I've been forced to address myself to the more important business at hand as I feud with the Boss. I meant it when I said I was lucky. I've lived on a higher plane than most, because it's the only unobstructed path. The garbage-strewn highways are not for me. Straight on—as the crow flies.

It's astonishing how clear things become when you stop smoking and fuming about bullshit. Not knowing *when* makes the *what* more important than the *why*. I may be more impatient than ever, but things get done and I only concern myself with good people who must be cherished, bad people who must be thwarted and my kids who must be spared the worst of me. There can't be enough laughter or the kind of great vibes that come from love.

I just don't have the time to waste on such popular time-wasters as jealousy, fools and envy. I was always too sure of myself for envy and jealousy, and truly do not begrudge enviable health in others. I love it and bask in it. It may even be catching. The only sin I do indulge in is greed. Greed for life, for every possible, extra-juicy funny moment. Since I've always wanted adventure and have to enjoy something, why not a house on the edge of a cliff? The suspense. Will he or won't he?

It's true that I watch family units wistfully and sometimes sting with sadness that it can never be my scene. But I do make cameo performances to some acclaim: Glenn and Gise, certainly, and their good friends Paul and Cathryn Brinkerhoff with their ten-year-old Jennifer, just as surely. Paul is six feet two and Thryn is up there, too. They're like a beautiful, new race or something.

"If Paul ever dies, we'll live together, Gary."

Shocked at what she had said, and responding to Paul's mock horror, she amended it. "I mean, of course, if he goes to Europe or something."

They're a wild and beautiful family, and when I visit in Connecticut, I indulge in my own fantasies that allow for hope. It's the same with my caring neighbors, Steve and Karin, and so many other happy couples I know. Of course, I'd like to share a life with someone else, one on one, if you'll forgive the image. I'd love to have my own kids; I'd really like that. Robin used to say that I'd make a great father. Anyway it's pointless, because it's my own decision.

If I ever really made the great move, I mean really reached out, it would be disaster time. If the woman came to love me, I feel I would only hurt her by failing, dying or worse. It would be the most immoral kind of seduction. So I've kept it light and airy and made impossible demands. If you insist on perfection, you've got it made and never lose control. She's going to fail and not me. It's so neat and so rotten.

I like to think that I've been forced into a semblance of nobility, but a secret part of me wishes, just for once, that I could turn what's left of my gaze to a pretty human curve, a lovely architectural angle, without first turning my back on the enemy. But I can't divide my attention. I've been told that I may be cheating that someone I'm so concerned about. Someone who *wants*, even *needs* to love me, but I can't allow myself such rationalization and her such philanthropy. A while back, did I say, "Let's wait until page 250?" Part of me wishes that I could be like everybody else and really court some particular darling who is bent on courting disaster (her problem I'm assured), but I can't. I guess I'm not like everybody else. Sue me.

There were several false alarms, notably March 1981, but surgery was again postponed because I wasn't ready. By December, there were a lot of loose ends to tie up, fences to mend. I had been on the alert for a year and a half, on blood transfusions for six months. I had one every two weeks for four months. No one can really tell me what those were all about. They had something to do with my antibodies, which allowed for a greater possibility of graft survival.

My own stupid blood could betray me just as that of my family, who couldn't be donors now for fear of being a kind of Trojan horse. My wonderful friends all came through with the usual cracks. "What do you want, my blood?" I certainly did. Debbie, Wendy, Mitchell—offers came from everywhere. But there still was no date, no time, no place for the actual event. The suspense was driving me crazy.

Up to the last moment, I reveled in what was left of my freedom. I could still dash off to New York or London (to everybody's distress) or Glenn and Gise's in Hartford or Bud Burton's in Carolina. There was almost a need to since I wasn't sure how soon I'd travel anywhere again. And Nancy, my oh so dependable driver, would take me anywhere I wanted to go around town. All of this was possible as long as I dotted my *t*'s and crossed my eyes.

At best, I would, for quite a while, be a slave to a machine and an unholy regimen. Subject to the scrutiny of doctors who would make Marge's "Have you tested?" sound like "Bon voyage, and don't bother to write, honey." Then there was always that possibility that it might not be such a *"bon"* voyage and maybe there'd be no news to write. No news wasn't such good news after all.

Up until the middle of January, I kept up my tennis, despite a dramatic diminution of energy. And I was certainly going to work every day. *At least I worked in a hospital—just in case,* I thought with a shiver.

There's always a crisis in the clinic, but there was a particularly tough fight I was having to see that Jose, a patient, was not sent to a home with a capital H, like the one in Hell. Maybe he did throw a few things at his "wicked stepfather." Jose was a bewildered, bitter kid who didn't want to be a hood but who didn't know what to do with his anger and his unnatural energy. Tell me about it!

His mother didn't want the burden of this terrified, curly haired fifteen-year-old. He was making it tough for her now that she was starting a new, seamy non-marriage. This street-wise innocent not only needed medical counseling but took up half my nights with sobbing phone calls pleading to be saved from institutionalization. The kid really had the book thrown at him.

While we both, at either end of the phone, medicated or supplemented our food intake to avoid trouble, I had the wee hours to solve an insoluble problem. Jose is emotional and desperate. Except for the frustrated and physically violent concern of an older brother, he is unloved. His mother has made her choice— the brutish SOB who is her new mate. I understand her, too. She's barely thirty. But I'm furious with her. She's a woman not a guppy. This is her kid.

Anyway, Jose would be better off in any home but his own at the moment, but the institution the social workers have recommended would transform this frightened, aggressive boy into a dying criminal. With his kept promise of cooperation and self-discipline plus better control of his diabetes, I was able to arrange

*251*

an interim period at a far better place totally acceptable to him. The point is that his phone calls are pleas for help. He wants to make it and he tries—the kid does, goddamn it, but he's always dodging brickbats. His disease, with its attendant demands, has not made him popular in the family.

There's no one he can talk to. So, question: How do you say, "It's four A.M., *amigo*. Go screw yourself?" Answer: You can't.

Being counselor to these clinic kids is something like being an AA sponsor to a "pigeon." They find you no matter where you are. I'll never refuse a call. I've even spoken with Jose and others while preparing for surgery. Their problems come first, of course.

That was another problem. My operation was more frightening to my patients than to me. First, there's the dependence and then the identification. I wanted to get the goddamned thing over with. Enough with cliff-hanging. There was too much that had to be done with the kids.

The days were dwindling down to a precious few. But I could still make decisions. Should I go to the Dolphins game at the Orange Bowl or play a little—very little—tennis? Should I take Wendy to lunch or how about calling Mitchell, or go for broke at the best Italian restaurant? Should I hang around my parents' pool and listen to some music or maybe plan another piece? I seemed to be slacking off in that department. How remarkable to have options even for a little while. I could still fly up to Hartford to see the bare trees and feel the snap of the cold air.

Ordinary people don't know the wonder of obeying a whim, satisfying an immediate need. Even going into the other room to raid the fridge. I was about to lose my autonomy and, before I did, I was going to run and be in five places at once. I was still beating the odds. Fooling them all. I saw the hostages return from Iran, the United States beat the Ruskies at hockey. I kissed the bride at Glenn's wedding and survived another election, which was more than some candidates did. I was still in there.

Toward the end of October, I flew up to New York with my parents and rendezvoused with Gise and Glenn so we could all attend the first annual Pisart Vision luncheon at the Plaza Hotel. I installed the original crystal sculpture, a copy of which is presented every year along with that fifteen thousand dollars to the winner. Marge and Marty, the whole gang was there—all thrilled with Orrefors' and Tiffany's execution of the piece. And so was I.

After wandering through the marvelous streets of New York and noting the progress of Philip Johnson's AT&T Building and then ogling the most beautiful girls in the world, who seem to have a permanent convention at Fifty-seventh and Fifth, we flew up to Boston to get the lay of the land at the hospital. Dr. Mintz wasn't sure as yet where the transplant would take place. Obviously I was plugging for all the men and women I knew down home and with whom I shared affection and respect. They *knew* me. At the sound of the bell, the whole team would jump to positions. But Dr. Mintz was not satisfied with the immunosuppressant, Imuran, that the University of Miami Hospital was forced to use. In Boston, the new Cyclosporin, evidently the more efficient, if experimental, drug, was his favorite and worth the New England trip.

It was discussable. The Miami staff that was involved with me personally was somewhat hesitant to have me be its first patient to use this new drug. Down home I could be victimized by their very concern and possible overprotection. In Boston the brand-new setup might challenge and alert me to all sorts of positive rewards. Dr. Mintz was preparing me for all contingencies, but he obviously wanted me to have this Cyclosporin rather than Imuran. It is now obvious that he had guided me away and eventually back to remove all doubt from my family's mind.

My respect for Boston's Joslin Clinic had grown with the years, and I came to recognize its unique and early-on, no-crap demand for Spartan control of diabetes. When I was a child, this approach was believed by many to make emotional cripples of the young. Despite this and my respect for the work done at Peter Bent Brigham Hospital in this charming, old town (charming old Carl Goldsmith was great enough to be there and sit in on the interview), I must frankly say that my enthusiasm for the home team remained undiminished after those interviews up there. "Why are you here?" one doctor asked me, though we had had the appointment for weeks. I guess I like being known, and longed for home. But I also wanted the best possible medication.

The dilemma was resolved and the decision not mine. Through Geneva's Dr. Albert Renold, a friend and colleague of Dr. Mintz, Cyclosporin was okayed officially in Miami. Everything had fallen or rather been shoved into place. It was now up to me. My count remained stable, even lowering somewhat as a tease.

Intuitively, Dr. Mintz knew that, despite these surprises, we were nearing the wire and last-minute preparations were made. It was then that my mother decided to visit with Glenn and Gise. She'd never taken a holiday—even for a couple of days—by herself; and she seemed to need to get away. She wanted to see Glenn and Gise and she had reason to want some space around her. She was going to return for her own surgery.

Yes, the chosen donor was my mother. If the reader has any sense of irony, he or she has already suspected as much. Marge's election by scientific tabulation was, I am convinced, aided by a lively campaign. My father's and my incredible rapport did not extend to the physical, and I know that my mother didn't relish having two sons with one kidney apiece.

Marge and I shared much more than our insufferable need to wash the soap and gild the lily. Kleiman versus Kleiman had turned into a merger.

Can you just imagine Them screaming with laughter up there. My mother, my lifelong antagonist. My mother, the woman I always feared was trying to castrate me. She would now actually control my functions. How could I ever again say, "Mom, will you get off my back?" She was there forever.

Marge's character, which has never been in any doubt, proved so sterling that now there was much more that I wished we had in common. The minute the decision had been made and our tissues as well as personalities were proved to be so similar, my mother started to bloom. She's not to be believed. Comforting my father, who was so worried about both of us, she simply said, "But, Marty, don't you see how wonderful it is to be able to give birth to him again?"

What was a guy supposed to do?

# 29

I T WAS THE GREAT switcheroo. I was visiting Marge in the hospital while she was taking some tests. It was bizarre seeing the boss lady lying there out of control. She was, of course, lovely to look at, calm and composed. But I knew from experience that I was seeing her for the first time beholden to others, vulnerable, dependent. She was also onstage and I was in the audience; and as with Glenn that time at Northwestern, I discovered how much worse it is to watch the sweep of a drama than it is to be the lead in it.

The horrendous effect my fucking chronicle was having on everybody else struck me more forcibly than ever. I couldn't stand seeing Marge in a hospital bed, following orders instead of giving them, lying down on the job. I knew what she must be feeling, and I hurt for her for the first time.

It also struck me that no matter her love and devotion and even some compensating need that might be satisfied by her sacrifice, she was giving me *part of her body*. It might have been noble and maternal but, goddamnit, it was unnatural. *Something could go wrong.* I had lived for ten years with the burden of my own mortality. But hers! This wasn't a tonsillectomy she was going to have. She was giving me a kidney. If something went wrong and she died, what would be the use of my being saved? Could anyone accept such a condition of survival? As with everything, we were going to give this our best shot, but if she died or anything, it would be the worst.

"You know," Marge said with that enraging reasonableness of hers, "it's no loss. We don't *need* two, which is fabulous, and the other kidney grows larger in compensation. Takes over all the work."

But we all get two when they're given out, and there must be a reason. I'm sure there isn't one extra in case a loved one needs it. I discussed this with Dr. Jacobs.

"I'd love to find evidence. I mean, someone who gave one and is still alive thirty years down the line."

"OK, you've got it. I'm the evidence."

"Thirty years? I remember now; you lost a kidney."

"As a matter of fact, it's *exactly* thirty years."

"It is?"

"Yeah, 1951."

"OK."

"And my remaining kidney hypertrophied so it's almost the size of two. You're not jeopardizing her longevity at all. Honest injun."

Well. All you've got to do is ask.

Although I kept worrying, there was no medical reason for doubting my mother wouldn't be all right. At forty-nine, she was in excellent health and, when those last tests were over, she truly anticipated the operation as lightly but dutifully as she would and did a Foundation underwriting luncheon.

Since those early, insecure days, Marge had become one of the great four-handkerchief money-raising speakers. But she'd run out of material and hated repeating herself. We all had decided, long ago over dinner, that my dying might attract donations dramatically, but we also recognized the overzealousness of such an approach. However! The oncoming surgery was an inspiration. My mother could stand there and ask for donations that—no matter how large—were but nothing compared to hers. Without that cure we were still waiting for, her son could no longer function. She was lucky enough to be able, if all went well, to renew

257

his lease on life. If, with the vast amount of money needed for research, the cure could be found during that time, this transplant and those people then would have really saved his life. She was confident, I was confident, and she swore standing there that in a matter of weeks both she and I would dance together at the annual Love and Hope Ball.

We have now, I pray, run out of catastrophes, but Marge was a sensation and the underwriting party a wild financial success. We raised a fortune that day. My feeling father, in an effort to spare the audience's sensibilities, would have stroked them. My mother aimed straight for the vein and it was the Comstock Lode. Thaddeus Foote, the president of the University of Miami, was so touched that he departed from his prepared address to say, "I have rarely been so touched, and have never heard a speech so heartfelt and elegant as Marge Kleiman's."

She now needed that rest up in Connecticut. The whole family had adjusted to the new script and was keeping it real light.

"You're flying, Mom? You must be kidding. Tell the pilot to keep his eyes open."

"Oh, my God. It never occurred to me, Gary. I won't go. I'll call them."

"Mom, I'm making like funny, you know? I trust Eastern. I fly it enough, but remember, you've got valuable cargo."

When she got there, she called to say that she arrived safely with her luggage and our kidney intact.

I think it was important that she see Glenn and Gise before the big day. Glenn, of course, didn't even want her to drive his car.

"Remember, Mom. You've got Gary's kidney to think of."

This woman had, like me, become a cliff-hanger. My body wouldn't send out the right welcoming message and neither my mother nor I knew for over a year whether in three days' time she would be under the knife, losing a kidney and possibly a son. You would never have known. First, because of her high spirits, and then by my own continuing one-sided battle with her. I had been programmed early and kept obeying obsolete directives.

258

Even her nobility was threatening to me. On one level, my admiration and gratitude could never be approximated, much less equaled. But in a sense, this was the battle I had always been fighting, and here it was in spades. The ultimate emasculation.

In my eyes, my mother was what she had always had to be—indispensable and at the controls. She was quite right when she said what she did. She *had* given me life and now she was renewing it. She *was* giving birth to me again. In some highly technocratic sense, she was simply and miraculously replaying her part in the natural scheme of things.

My mother's instincts have always been wholesome, springing as they do from some first reckoning. It's I who's the rebel gene, obviously imperfect, abrasive and demanding special maverick status: obeying my own impulses, cutting across the grain, forced to make my own, sometimes brash, rules concerning my own survival. Marge's emotional resources—annoyingly enough—even encompassed these. There's no measuring the woman.

For years my mother and I had that wall of steel between us. It's still a wall, but now it's cellophane, all the better to see each other clearly. What do you want? Only in fiction does revelation bring about a real about-face. We're both complicated people in a complicated relationship and more than usually and irrevocably attached.

Marty, my father—a mere man—couldn't ever accept my behavior, especially toward Marge. Now, he could only try to accept this new situation that threatened both his wife and son.

Once, long ago, when I was at my lowest at the Rice House, I asked Marty if he believed in God.

"I don't know," he answered. "I've never really asked him for anything before this. We'll see."

Knowing my father's high tolerance of wickedness and his irrational trust in humankind, I could only suspect, with this new crisis, that he was also going to give *Him* another chance. But I watched his smile get more frantic and his jokes cornier as the interminable wait was evidently coming to an end.

Debbie was giving me a transfusion in my office at the unit. Very informal as usual.

"When Mintz does give us a definite date, Glenn's going to throw up, Gise's going to cry and Dad's going to go crazy hysterical and have sweaty hands. Really, Deb, the wrong people are playing the leads. The tough ones are participating and the worst ones are watching. Marge and I could handle it much better."

"You've both got enough to handle. It's getting real close, Gar. The last creatinine was six point four."

"Jesus, what basketball I could have played from that height."

"You're a scream."

"Yeah, in the night."

"I don't think it's going to be·too long."

"I know. I'm nauseous a lot. I can't eat. I feel shitty. But not *real* shitty, you know? Well, Deb, you actually found the vein."

"Screw yourself, sugar."

"Can't you see I'm busy at the moment?"

"You'll feel real bad in a short time. Then you'll be just fine."

"Yeah." I paused. "He died, didn't he?"

"Who?"

"George Washington. What do you mean, 'who'?"

"Oh, you mean Tom Whats'isname?"

"Oh, I mean Tom Whats'isname? What really happened?"

"That was an entirely different story, Gar, and I don't really know. It was a real terrible thing, and it was the partial pancreas business not the kidney that went wrong during the operation. It was peritonitis."

"That's encouraging, and where will Dr. Elmer T. Butterfingers be on T day? I hope nowhere near me."

"You've got the best, and it's all different."

"Yeah. You know, Gise asked about Tom yesterday."

"She did?"

"I was talking to Connecticut. I wanted to know how Glenn was handling all this now that it's on top of us. And she just asked."

"Did you tell her?"

"I couldn't *not*, but I hated to. You know they've only heard the good things, that no one's come out of a transplant with as much as a hiccup. Now he's dead, the kid."

"But so many others aren't."

"That's not what Glenn and Gise are going to remember. It's Tom, *not* the others. Just when they were getting it all together."

"Gar, you know I don't con you. You're not going in to have a tooth pulled, but you can die having a tonsillectomy, too."

"Somehow I'd prefer risking that. . . . I heard Tom's blood sugar went to six hundred. I mean, that's like crazy. You know, just for a split second—less than that maybe, I'm going to be a little anxious. You know, scared."

"What's the big deal? You're only losing kidneys."

"Don't worry. I'll put on my S cape and—watch out."

"Now that's the Gary I know and envy. Invulnerable."

"That's the Gary everybody knows. Sometimes I wonder but just for moments."

"Honey, the last transplant now has a creatinine of one point four."

"It's been a long time. One point four—I'm getting sentimental over you."

"Remember, Gar, when we all, when I particularly was so into *quality* of life? Well I'm into quantity now."

Debbie looked at me hard.

"And I do mean it. You should have seen the other guy, the other transplant's face when I told him 'one point four.' I haven't heard one complaint yet from one of those guys. I swear."

"You've sold me, Deb. I'm looking forward to it. I'm free tomorrow afternoon. How about it?"

Wendy walked into the office and fell into a chair.

"Where are we going tomorrow? Let's split and have a bite or a movie or something. . . . Is that the last transfusion Deb is giving you?" she asked.

"Yeah." Debbie bent my arm. "Thanks, Deb. It's been a thrill. Really, Wendy, it's so great like this, doing it myself."

"*I* thought I was here."

"I mean with Debbie. It's a helluva lot smoother than when they do it. I mean, look. I organized the whole transfusion, and if Deb couldn't, I had Maria ready as a backup. The donated blood also had a backup ready and was washed and delivered by twelve. Perfect. Done. Finished. Nothing to it and Deb is a dream."

"Thanks, hon."

"You know, I came over—it's funny—I wanted—don't object now or get all hung up," Wendy sputtered.

"Out with it."

"I wanted to feel sorry for you."

"Go right ahead. I'm in the mood."

"I can't. I was on my way over thinking, 'Enough already. The guy's had it.' We need you here at the unit and I thought of how scared you must be and then here you are, insufferable as ever."

"Great, isn't it?"

"No. I *want* to feel sorry for you and you won't let me."

"You remind me of a girl I was seeing once."

"Once only?"

"Not much longer. We weren't getting anywhere and she said, 'Good! I don't have to put up any walls. You already have yours.' "

"That's sad," Debbie said.

"No, it's not. It's ridiculous."

"You're a riot, Gary."

"That's me all over."

"How can you even banter with everything so close?"

"I'm not being gung ho. It just isn't real. That's the truth."

"But it is and it's OK. It's funny. Everybody—all the doctors here—is so really optimistic. No, I mean it. Kyriakides, Miller, Mintz, Skyler, everybody. Because it's *you* probably and because you're so damned indestructible and because it—well—it just, it just looks good."

"I remember asking, months ago, what would happen if they open Mom up and she only had one kidney? *That* was going to be a real test of mother love! Would she or wouldn't she? I told her, 'You know, Mom, what I always say, quality *must be* tested.' "

"What did *Marge* say?"

"She told me if I got too fresh she'd change her mind and not give me any at all."

"Great."

"Using the old reward technique. Marge is terrific."

"Yeah. But if anything happened to her under the knife or—well, you never know, do you? I couldn't live with that. I mean, what would be the point?"

"Nothing is going to happen, Gary. She's in great shape."

"That's right, doll. Your Mom will be just fine, and you know what Mintz said. She really wants this; she really wants to do this. It's important to her. You're allowing her to—"

"Look, guys. I'm OK. Don't give me all this. The whole thing isn't real. It's not my life anyway, so what's the difference? Like I'm supposed to feel awful, really awful, and I really don't feel like I'm dying."

"You're not. You're just getting a kidney transplant."

"Right. But if I wasn't, I'd be dying."

"I guess so. It's interesting."

"It depends on where you're standing. How much deterioration can I take? Not to the kidneys—they're gone already—but other things. How regenerative—"

"You'll be all right, honey. The unit wouldn't be the unit without all three of us. So when it's over, we expect you to get those little buns out of bed fast."

"Right. Debbie says that the success rate is very high."

"That's so, sugar."

"Right. But I was thinking, it's all so terrific until I realize the details. I mean the bare facts. They're going to take Mom's kidney out, wash it off and slap it into me. Think about it. It's wild—a small mistake, even an itty-bitty one—"

"There is no way they are going to make a mistake. Everybody's watching. The JDRF, the press and all the frustrated women in your life."

"Including us, hon."

"Anyway, it's almost here, guys. You know, we've been talking months, then weeks, now days, and then it'll be hours and then it'll be *it*. T day, and then it'll be yesterday, and then weeks ago, then months and oh, I hope, years. I feel the future brushing past me."

On the alert for six years, I had been hearing that drumroll for eighteen months. Then suddenly it was here. The countdown. Three, two, one, zero hour."

"Gary has a date," Wendy announced in the office one day.

"Who with?" Debbie asked. "Do I know her?"

Gary had a date all right. With his mother, Dr. Kyriakides, my surgeon, and Dr. Miller, hers. A double date. Rain or shine, sick or healthy, ready or not, it was definitely set for January 20, 1982.

The unbelievable was coming to pass and the reality was dizzying and grotesque. A sense of urgency unrelated to specifics sent me spinning. I called everyone I knew to spread the news and went ahead with Marge and Marty to give the party we had been planning all along. I thought seriously of sending kidney-shaped notes but settled for invitations that just asked all our close friends to a pre-opening dinner and gala at our house for January 16, which was a Saturday night. Marge and I were to enter the hospital on Sunday.

The party was important to me. It was to be a kind of roundup of all the guys I loved, everyone I've been writing about. I wanted to share laughter and life with them one more time before who knew what. We love celebrations in my family and this was a real lulu. A doubleheader. Glenn and Gise, my grandparents, friends, loves, doctors, lawyers, beggar men, colleagues, a real gathering of the clan. Everybody accepted and Dr. Jacobs had some fears for me.

"But it'll be a ball," I said. "Having the whole cast singing and dancing. I don't get the point."

"But, Gary, what happens after the ball is over and the masks are dropped at twelve o'clock? When everybody remembers why there was a party at all?"

Dr. Mintz wasn't sure about the bash either, for about the same reasons.

"But, Dan, they've been looking forward to this so much," my father said.

"It'll be great," I insisted. "Mom and I will leave them laughing. You'll see."

Both doctors were afraid that, along with the dirty dishes and tired balloons, a deflated, bedraggled Gary would be part of the debris. After all, under the circumstances, how do you say, "Good night, what a great time, see you around?" They needn't have worried.

From first to last, it was a beautiful night and bursting at the seams with loving people. I may be selective and demanding in my relationships, but I've got the greatest friends on this planet. We had sixty guests and there wasn't one single asshole. There was a lot of hugging and kissing and I like that. There was so much laughter and a lot of nice crying. The kind you see at weddings.

Everybody descended on our Bay Road house like crazy angels. I mean, everybody I cared about was there. It was like a coda of a symphony. All the themes and motifs becoming one in a crash of cymbals. Not that I needed proof, but it was really nice to know how much they all cared about us. Everybody was right on and no one bothered to hide his emotions. I loved it.

I think, too, that it was a release from tension. The threatening storm had broken and the rains had come. The general feeling was that they wouldn't flood and destroy but nourish and replenish.

It was certainly a sentimental evening. What else? Old buddies Jeff Arthur and Rod Glaubman brought their guitars and played songs we'd written together and everybody sang—and danced. I remember thinking, *When I feel a little stronger, I'll have a good cry about all of this.* It was great.

My father was a baronial host, my mother radiant and I was,

as always, a blue streak with a red beard. Early on, I started having a reaction—possibly because of all the excitement—and was therefore the first to attack the terrific buffet. Then I was OK. I reveled and really basked in all the sunniness. And quite late, the really close, great people—you know, the wonderful dregs—stayed on and on; and I thought that it had better be only the seventh inning. And if it was really the ball game, then what a way to go.

"Are you really going to show up for this thing Wednesday?" Wendy asked.

"I haven't decided. I love last-minute decisions."

"Well, remember, you'll be charged anyway."

I watched Marge being both hostess and honored guest with her usual style and it hit me again. This time with a real wallop. I was used to facing the unfaceable, the edge of a volcano was my natural habitat, strong medicine my daily diet. I no longer reeled from all of this, I swaggered. But my mother, electively, was walking into the hospital with me—to stay. I mean, my mother *chose* to go under the knife of her own free will—for me. She wasn't sick; she was perfect and she was going to have these men futz around with her insides. She thought of it gaily as a simple subtraction, but I was never good at arithmetic or math and I only understood one thing. If anything happened to Marge, there was no hell terrible enough for me.

# 30

I PRECEDED MY MOTHER into the hospital by a day. There was much more rigmarole attached to my part of the act. In the first place, they had to start my newly approved but still-mysterious drug, Cyclosporin. My first dose was massive and I reacted like a woman in menopause. Hot flashes kept me in a perpetual blush. My wrists and neck were on fire and I really felt like a rapidly charring sacrifice to the cloud sitters. If I was, I hoped I'd give them all heartburn.

It wasn't possible to make too much sense because the drug really spaced me out. Voices and faces were receding swiftly, psychedelically. It seems that Cyclosporin's booster steroid, Medrol, which is insulin-resistant, was sending my sugar to the moon. My usual insulin dosage was now trebled, but my sugar remained measurable not in numbers but in grocery-store pounds. The obvious insult to my body was throwing everything out of whack. To make absolutely certain that the drama not sag, there was, out of nowhere, a lot of talk about factor eleven, my blood's inability to coagulate. The usual count for coagulation is forty-one. I wasn't getting it all together until sixty-two. I didn't have enough on my mind without that. *It must be the alpine sugar,* I deduced, conjectured or fantasized in an effort to consult with my doctors. I wasn't giving up my consultant status ever.

Frozen plasma was brought in the second day and that's all I was on. Liquids and the cold stuff. I couldn't help but think how socially acceptable Dracula would be today, satisfying his desperate needs at the Board of Health or some medical supermarket instead of resorting to all that antisocial jazz. It would do wonders for his personality.

Mine had seen better days. On the afternoon of my second day, I was hooked up with lines and wires until I looked like a Rube Goldberg drawing. Everything I owned was attached to something. There were extensions all over the place. This main line—the Atchison, Topeka—originated down south someplace and, moving under the collarbone, terminated in the large cardiac artery and continuously fed me calories and insulin.

Marge and I had a hot line between our rooms. She was in the process of improving the service in the hospital and rehanging the pictures. We were both going through endless tests and she was whizzing through them, getting high marks on all. I was failing one after another. Every bit of news was a headline.

Up to the day before surgery, there was suspense. There had been a cancellation of the same operation a week before because of sudden incompatibility. There was a possibility this could have happened to my mother and me. The tissue tests were repeated daily. We got the final "it's go" on the eve of the operation.

It was then discovered that I had a positive surface antigen of serum hepatitis. This meant that either I had had the disease without knowing it or it was on its merry way. In any case, though it was dormant, Kyriakides and any other member of the operating team who came into contact with my blood, could contract the disease. What a reward for their work! I could break out with it at any moment and start an epidemic. Would this delay surgery? *Could* surgery be delayed? I was, you remember, now sick enough.

The recital of calamities and near fatalities had lost its power to thrill. I listened with half an ear, no longer able to absorb all the implications. I later heard that Marge, on hearing of this new snag, lost her cool for a moment and shouted, "Damn them! Haven't they done enough to my boy?" We would see.

Now that I was in the big time, I had to be properly groomed, so they came in and shaved every goddamned thing I own except my beard. Then came the real class act—the enemas. I was purged, cauterized, made immaculate and scared shitless. For good measure, all of this was followed by Betadine baths. I was now as spotless and germ-free as my mother's kitchen. Actually, at this point, I was numb. In a very short while, my life was going to be totally in the hands of others. I would be helpless, my eagle eye unable to seek out and avert danger. I was relinquishing control—the dreaded nightmare. Dr. Kyriakides briefed me. I didn't want any surprises—except good ones. He told me pretty much what to expect: a three-hour operation unless something went wrong on my mother's side, then a catheter to remove my body fluids, since the kidney, like any transplanted life, would be in shock and not in great working order. *Unless something went wrong.*

I got the gags ready just in case. The whole shtick was filed away neatly. I realized how much like my mother I was. *That's to the good,* I thought. *That's terrific.* Wouldn't that mean the kidney would be truly compatible?

While I was worrying about all this, the phone didn't stop and I realized how many people were depending on me. Not only my family and friends who loved me and my army of doctors who for more far-reaching reasons wanted me to emerge the victor, but my patients who really needed me. I'd also been trying to get a dear and troubled friend in New York into proper medical hands. I really couldn't afford to be out of commission long. Above all, the kids were on my mind, especially little Kevin, five years old and starting on insulin—so sweet the mosquitoes won't leave him in peace.

Kevin is a precious child who lets me share his awful sugar-free cookies and makes a toy of the white cap that protects his syringe. Brand new and seemingly untouched, his sunny face dissolved into that of an emaciated old man as I lay drugged and half-dreaming.

*I've got to write that book. I don't want Kevin to lie here someday, a human switchboard.*

Glenn and Gise were staying with my father, who was certainly going to need them. Marge was worried about them all.

"Everything is just fine. When you see me, it'll be all over and we'll both be great. Look, the linens were changed, there's some beef in the fridge and, please, get Dad out to a picture or something tonight."

My mother was never for a moment anything but optimistic. We had the best doctors, the best intentions and the best friends in the world plugging for us. All the vibes were perfect, so there was no question in her mind.

Nonetheless, I had my routine of jokes just in case her sacrifice was pointless. I really wanted to let her know. I prayed it wouldn't come to that, but I was ready.

"I swear, Mom. There's nothing personal about this. I'm not rejecting you again." And stuff like that there.

There *was* that possibility. Tests or no tests, when it came to the moment of truth, my cocky, stubborn body just might fight this latest invasion of privacy. Who knew? The only alternative would be the dreaded dialysis. The rest was not discussable.

Dr. Mintz spoke with me at this point. Holding my hand, he called me his friend. He assured me that there was every reason to believe in the complete success of the operation. Everything had fallen into place and the entire team was raring to go.

He believed this, but he is a scientist and a realist. His reading was carefully understated, allowing for error, the capricious, the mystery ingredient. I translated his message and it was good enough. I saw his earnestness, knew how carefully everything had been planned, was well aware of my surgeon's gifts. There was a kind of white light—a blaze of good energy—from everyone, including our friends.

270

I submitted to my doctors with much more than blind faith.

The shots were taking effect and I was half-asleep as they wheeled me down to the operating room. I knew my way around this hospital. I'd raced and strutted through most of it and now felt humiliated entering elevators and corridors feet first, facing the ceilings. It was really like a movie with the camera taking the place of the actor. What a view, lying there, sliding along disgustingly on display, subject to the rude and curious gaze of visitors and the bored disregard of much of the medical staff.

As the nurse maneuvers a bed into an elevator, the interns or whoever reflexively move their butts to accommodate it, but evidently forget what's on it—for instance, people with ears.

"Where are you coming from, Tim?"

"Number three. The Simpson dame—cardiac arrest before they could even touch her liver. How about lunch when I'm cleaned up?"

I know what elevator small talk can be like in hospitals and I prayed I wouldn't hear my name or Marge's. I might have been made privy to the odds for my survival.

The nurse made a sharp turn down one of the halls and I was surprised to find myself in a holding room. *Jesus, something else has gone wrong; if there's another delay, I'll go ape.*

"What's wrong, nurse?" I asked groggily.

"Nothing. You're going to meet an old friend."

There was a kind of green paper shower curtain dividing the room, and when it was pulled away, I saw my mother—a mirror image of me—in a green surgical gown and cap. But for the change in uniform, she was still the general on the way to battle, ready to direct the entire operation, even under anesthesia.

Despite her smile, her face was so white that I half-believed that she'd already been to surgery and was on her way back, her kidney floating around the building, having been rejected by others beside myself. My heart really missed a beat. But this was

271

only my mother without makeup. She had always said—and now I knew why—that without the necessary goo, she looked like a discard from Forest Lawn.

"Hi!"

"Hi!"

"Ready?"

"I'm sleepy."

"Do good," she said gaily, using the family toast.

"OK."

During the pre-opening party, my mother and I had thought that it might be a great idea if we increased the chances of compatibility, actual oneness, if we went under the knives thinking the same thing, sharing the same frequency. We were hard put to decide on what it would be. Wildly, she had suggested snappers.

"I can't get an image. I don't even know what the hell they look like."

"OK, what about a parrot? Let's think of a parrot."

"Great. A gorgeous green parrot."

"Red, Gary. I see a red parrot. We'll mess it up."

"What about black bowling balls?"

"Perfect," my mother had said.

Now her eyes brightened in the holding room.

"Remember, darling. Black bowling balls. Hold the image."

"Right. Black bowling balls."

"It'll be a breeze."

"No sweat."

"Do good."

"You, too. See you later."

The smart-ass talk was over and we were soon in the hands of pros. In three hours' time, my mother's beautiful, healthy kidney was washed and cradled into my right hip, because my own kidneys were left in place to atrophy. It was, as they say, a textbook case, a perfect performance by all.

I was really out of it when I returned to some form of consciousness. I felt every single tube invading my body, and I heard lots of commotion. I didn't even have the energy or desire to open my eyes to see what was going on. Cutting through the blur of sounds was Debbie's drawl. "Isn't he going to open his eyes?"

"I don't think so," a muffled, unidentifiable voice answered.

The urgency in Debbie's voice and her subsequent gasp dragged me back to the land of the living. I roused myself and could just about make out Deb and a lot of other people in green caps and gowns and masks. I must have smiled or something because crazy Debbie became radiant.

"Welcome, honey," she said. "It was perfect."

For someone who has raced through the years and not always demonstrated his feelings, those days just before and after surgery were highly emotional. Tears were always near the surface, and any sign of caring, of concern for me or my mother touched a foot pedal that made my water fountain gush. I mean, I was crying at dog food commercials.

There were sixty people in the waiting room for those three hours and not one of them was able to control my father, who was possessed as he waited for Dr. Meitus's bulletins personally delivered every half hour. Glenn and Gise didn't leave his side, which made them all crazy. When one of the bulletins was a couple of minutes late, my father went raving into the halls. I don't know how they all survived. I knew the wrong ones were watching.

My mother, for all her elegance, is obviously a peasant. Within ten hours of surgery, she was feeling fine and her only medication was Demerol. The next morning, though still in some discomfort, she refused all drugs and was given some nonnarcotic, synthetic analgesic named Stadol. After that, she was on nothing but Extra-Strength Tylenol. But we know what she must have gone through. Glenn, by this time reporting for NBC, told me that when he first saw Marge after the operation, he could only think of the day he covered Ella Grasso's funeral in Hartford. "I swear, Gar, the governor looked better that day than Mom."

But my mother is durable, too. As for her education in

humor, she's graduated summa cum laude. Just as she was about to go under, she said to the anesthetist, "You know, having a baby is easy. It's the maintenance that's tough." Brilliant. And she said it and then just closed her eyes. Real timing. If she developed that under my tutelage, I learned breeding from her.

My room was filled with flowers and fruit and gifts from everywhere, including The Lighthouse. I would eventually acknowledge them. I wasn't quite ready for such a list, but I made a start. My first note was delivered to her room as soon as I was able to write.

> Dear Mom,
> I want to thank you for your generous gift. It fits, it works and, honestly, it was exactly what I needed.
>> Love,
>> Gary

When Marge was, at last, allowed to leave her room, she insisted on seeing me to make sure our telephone exchanges weren't setups. I don't think she believed I was still around. Still, when she got the OK to come to my room, she practically went to Elizabeth Arden first. Gise claims that my mother wouldn't see me until she was presentable and healthy looking. That was fine with me, considering the shock I'd experienced seeing her in that holding room.

I, too, wanted to look my best to alleviate any fears she might have had, but there wasn't too much I could do, I was attached to so many parts of the building. I wonder how much of this was sensitivity or just plain old vanity.

My chair was near the window when Marge was wheelchaired over to me. She looked terrific in a new, red dressing gown and she was in full, glorious technicolor makeup—all of this under the necessary mask. It was insane. She looked like a near-eastern spy or maybe Gina Lollobrigida posing as a patient in a dubbed Italian movie called *The Great Hospital Heist*. I half-expected her to remove a pearl-handled pistol from under her kerchief. She really looked great. The entire scene was bizarre, the plot line unacceptably unrealistic.

274

We didn't say a word and just stared at each other, and then Marge burst into tears.

"Oh, I'm sorry, Gary. I swore I wouldn't do this. I tried."

But I almost blew my tubes I was so choked up. We reached out through all the wires and lines and bottles, through all the shit and all the years, and for the first time since my babyhood, we clung to each other, my mother and I. We clung to each other for dear life.

# 31

I WAS HOLDING my own and everybody was holding his breath. But on Day Five, my creatinine count started to go haywire and there was real concern. Could I be rejecting? The numbers were fluctuating perilously. What was happening is called ATN, acute tubular necrosis, and I voyaged down from my room on my first postoperative trip to get a renal scan.

A minute amount of radioactive dye was injected and the area of the kidney then closely observed. It was quickly discovered that the erratic behavior of the kidney was caused either by the lack of oxygen caused by its hazardous spattering transposition from Marge to me—or the Cyclosporin.

At any rate, now with terrible gas pains gone and concentrating on this book and its beginnings, I refused to be agitated by the numbers game. I had, after all, seen trees and plants first languish then flourish after relocation. There was no question that the congenial environment and devoted care of this newcomer could cushion its shock and homesickness, but I am thoroughly convinced that its desire to live and thrive is a prime factor. I've seen plants give up too, and I've seen people do the same, some even subsisting in defeat, half-caring. I could never do that. If you're going to stick around then, damnit, you fight like hell.

Toward the end of the first week I felt a little stronger but disappointed that the ATN was still fluttering so. I was looking a bit more human once the venal line had been removed. The catheter remained, however. It was my only artificial extension now, but it was enough. My trips to other parts of the hospital by wheel proved to be the worst aspect of the postoperative period. Gary, the wheeler and dealer, being wheeled around always mortified me. Again, it's worst in the elevators.

"What a young man. Has a heart condition?" a woman asked as if I weren't there.

"How kind of you to be concerned," I answered sweetly.

The renal scan isn't fun, and I'm never in the best mood when I'm about to have one. I thought of the kids at the unit. If only they could be spared all this crap.

And, still, my luck held. A very nice guy who had been on dialysis for two years and had just had a transplant from a cadaver didn't make it. The kidney was working but his heart gave out. Another transplanted young lady hadn't survived subsequent surgery for complications either. I was furious I wasn't told about these failures immediately. In addition to Tom—the guy Debbie told me about—the terrible information should have depressed me. But the law of averages applies even to death. The SOB is always hanging around hospitals. He likes hospitals and has many willing helpers there. Nevertheless, I felt encouraged. I figured that I was the guy who was going to make it.

Now I was becoming toxic. My whole family is sensitive, both positively and negatively, to medications. A smidgen can do the trick or make us ill, since we all react to everything. When I told the doctors this, that a mere whisper of something foreign and I'd salute, they started to diminish the dosages.

Some literature was delivered to me—a book called *The Better Life*, apparently designed to reach the simple and pure of heart. We readers were to believe that the rest of the diabetes work load, now augmented by daily Cyclosporin, the exact amount of which has still to be determined, plus another fistful of must's, constituted a life made better. It is now necessary to take my temperature every single day. If it goes above one hundred degrees, there's a special number I must call. If my weight varies, either way, by more than two pounds, there's another emergency number.

There were so many new rules to my book of regulations that I actually dreamed one night that I decided not to have the transplant since it was far too much trouble. But I awakened with my usual compulsions.

I was still bargaining on my subconscious to back up my fight. Down deep in the lowliest root of my being, I prepare for the next round. Confiding this to Wendy on Day Seven, when even He was allowed to rest, my sugar had risen to five hundred and the creatinine was soaring. The miraculous drug that was specially dispensed to me might prove to be my undoing. There was talk of switching medications.

Wendy reminded me that nothing was endless and every time I had had a crisis that seemed terminal I had prevailed.

"Then you will," Barbara had said to me.

So many people have faith in me. So many people expect the impossible, and I keep delivering. They make me feel I can do it, and I'm my own best press agent besides. Still, after the transplant I discovered that even the strong need replenishment to keep them strong. I will never again think that anyone—least of all me—can function alone, apart, independent of others. I will never again not celebrate the fact that this need to share and satisfy our resources is as strong and pervasive as the individual's clawing instinct for survival.

More than ever, I thought of my kids, of the looks on their faces when they are presented with the unavoidable restrictions and duties that will interrupt their lives incessantly and make them subject to such negative attention. The boringness of it. The unrelieved, smashing, clobbering boringness of such self-indulgence. How can we avoid becoming egomaniacs?

Those terrible days in the hospital I thought that if I could somehow, with the help of all my doctors, truly welcome Marge's kidney, make it feel at home, if I could get out of the damned place in working order and, in simplest terms, cleanse myself of impurities, that I would work harder than ever. If I had a few more years, at least I would dig in and make the necessary labor more vivid and fun for my patients. As an old vet, I'd managed to integrate all the jazz into a life worth living. And I did want to live. Damnit, life is a feast, and despite my diet, my table manners and the garbage that pursues banquets, I'll take it all. I don't even have a choice. It's my rubber ass Edna Glaubman bequeathed to me. But Christ, even Jesus with the fourth nail said, "Enough already!" He really did, only the King James Version translated it as, "Oh, Lord, why hast thou forsaken me?"

It was touch and go for quite a while, and I scribbled notes on lined yellow legal paper, carefully, almost detachedly, keeping a log with notes for this book.

*Day Eight*

Danger of rejection is great. Sugar is still rising. Creatinine is up to 4.6, my BUN 112. Shit! Feeling dopey and weak. Headache—obviously autointoxicated. Spoke to little Kevin. Can't wait to see him.

*Day Nine*

They won't believe it about my sensitivity to medication. Plan to cut my Cyclo in half. Even Dr. Mintz seems puzzled and dejected. "Be patient," they're all saying. I'm just the guy. They roll me in and out. I feel like a carpet.

*Day Ten*

Stabilized. Feel great. Dreamed I was still trying to postpone surgery. Too late!

*Day Eleven*

Creatinine going down slowly. Exhausted. Marty looks terrible. Know they're all crossing their fingers. I have news, so am I. Mom going home. Great! One to go.

*Day Twelve*

Planning another renal scan and biopsy. Feeling better but numbers stopped coming down. It took fifteen years for *my* kidneys to go. What the hell is the ATN doing to this expectancy?

*Day Thirteen*

Am concentrating on 3.9. I *will* get it below 4—if it *kills* me.

Got to get rid of all the sludge. This kidney's going to work—or else. When Dr. Mintz visits, he stays until my need is satisfied or problem resolved. What a guy.

*Day Fourteen*

*The worst happened,* I thought. My eye blurred and then went totally blind except for brilliant flashes of light and bands of gorgeous color. I was terrified, so was my father, so was the nurse and so was Dr. Mintz. I was having my own private horror show. Screamed bloody murder and I wish Carl Goldsmith wasn't sick himself and was here. The rest think it was a reaction to urinary medication. It was the worst yet, but it passed. Sight returned later in the day along with heartbeat and hope.

*Day Fifteen*

Am down to 2.09. How about that? Looks good. Hope to be out of here in a few days. Heard the doctors talking in hall. Are they using mikes? I'm still not out of danger. Screw them.

*Day Sixteen*

Wall Street Report. Sugar and BUN down. Creatinine steady. Hopes high and future's looking up.

*Day Seventeen*

The human yo-yo. Need transfusion and Dr. Mintz promised me specific donorship. Wendy, Debbie, friends—no strangers. Count up again and Kyriakides debating new biopsy. Am taking in tremendous amount of fluid and peeing like there's no tomorrow. Oops! Shut yo' mouth. Biopsy dangerous because of my factor eleven. Am not clotting quickly enough. Lovely!

*Day Twenty-two*

February 11. *Home!* We're still futzing around with numbers, but as the song goes, "I'm still here" and feeling fine. It's great being home, although the place looks like a nest of bandits—everyone in protective masks. Had a great turkey sandwich and tried running upstairs. No way. An Australian crawl is more like it. Marvelous to be in my own bed with nobody annoying me.

I've been thinking of kidney-shaped structures and pools. I wonder why. And that makes me think of Henry Moore and that makes me think of Mom's kidney tucked in my hip cavity which makes me think of the master's interlocking forms. I mean, it's unbelievable. I *am* a bloody Henry Moore.

Must tell Sandy that I tried jumping today as if I were making a basket back in Syracuse and couldn't even get off the ground. It was like a dream. You know, like trying to flee and being glued to the spot. Got to do something and soon. The Foundation ball is not too far off. It would be a great finish for the book.

We keep our promises in our family. On February 20, exactly one month after the transplant, Thaddeus Foote, the president of the University of Miami, announced to the five hundred applauding guests in the Hotel Diplomat's ballroom that Marge Kleiman and her son Gary would lead the dancing. Are you ready? The orchestra played *"Margie"* as my mother and I stepped out on the floor and whirled around in a spotlight. I loved it. It was the height of corniness and if we weren't exactly Fred Astaire and Ginger Rogers, everybody loved it—from Governor Bob Graham to the busboys. If all the lights had blown, there would still have been the glare and radiance of my father's grin to light our way.

More and more couples joined us on the dance floor and I heard Glenn and Gise's laughing voices as we brushed past them. All I could make out in the crazy light were the colors and shapes of wonderful people who had been part of my life forever and, without doubt, were to varying degrees responsible for my being there. I was kind of drunk on the miracle of it all. What my mother and the doctors and all these caring people had done could never be summed up or properly esteemed in a speech or tribute or even a book.

When we were passing our table, Marty Kleiman, the new president of the JDRF, cut in to dance with his wife and at the same time delicately see to it that I wasn't overdoing it. That was impossible. My parents drifted off in their wonderful oneness and, in a kind of revelation, I saw the whole ballroom that way. Both my vision and emotional state made a beautiful blur of all these individuals. In a kind of epiphany, I knew how I'd survived, and the only way the rest of the world could survive. By being part of each other, or giving and sharing love and hope. The ball was well named.

It was one of those moments, perhaps feverish or ecstatic or delirious, when everything falls into place and in a terrible clarity you know that, if there isn't any order or design, then we must make it ourselves. That if there are no gods, then we must become them. My family, my friends, my saviors, my kids and my art all became one.

With total recall, I saw Barbara Hepworth's garden. The tranquil green, the pieces still there, her immortality. All of us part of the landscape. In a kind of madness, I thought that even disease in trees, in plants is conquered eventually, is even—if you're not of the particular species—lovely to the eye. Art was only a method of rearranging particulars and celebrating life. Barbara had said that, at all times, under any condition, art should be an act of praise and sensibility to the oneness of man and his landscape.

I've always done what I could, trusting to nothing less than efficiency, but I'm well aware that without luck, you can forget it. I've been lucky in many things, beginning with my choice of family.

I'm hanging in there. It was always my contention that, not knowing from day to day what was going to happen, it was difficult for me to plan. If I were certain of five years, I would intensify. If I were certain of ten, I would be able to make a real commitment. That was before the transplant and my convalescence and my working on this, my story.

A truck, for Christ's sake, can hit anybody, and I'm filled with better vibes than I've ever had. Despite the intelligence that my new kidney is just a new lease on a shaky life, that the old diabetes has already started to destroy it along with everything else I've got, I also know how mysterious the life force is and how facts can be altered or absolutely replaced by legend.

I'm ready to intensify and I'm ready to commit myself. In all

282

departments. I feel I have even more to offer my kids since the operation. I feel rededicated to my art through my recognition of its positive appraisal and improvement of life. There are two new commissions possible—one for Dadeland Metrorail Complex that is really exciting.

Judie and I were supposed to spend Halloween 1982 in New York with Glenn and Gise. I wanted to see the Empire State Building all orange and red and prepared to duck flying broomsticks! I wanted to see Greenwich Village turn into New Orleans with its crazy parade of witches, saints and irreverent observers and, of course, to take another look at Barbara's single form at the United Nations. Unfortunately, Judie had a cold so we couldn't fly. But we're planning on making the trip soon, I can hardly wait.

Now hear this. My kid brother Glenn has just, at NBC-Hartford, received two Emmy nominations—for investigative and in-depth reporting. How about that? He will get one of them. I know it.

Dr. Kyriakides definitely wants to take a triple scan and an ultrasound again this next week. He's put off the biopsy for a while. I trust it won't keep me from flying up to Boston. It's just for the weekend, of course, since my clinic work is full time again.

Yesterday I asked little Kevin the question I ask all my patients, no matter his or her age. "What do you like most about yourself, Kevin? Tell me."

Kevin is really something else. He screwed up his face and thought very hard. "I'm a good boy," he answered.

"That's what everybody else likes about you, Kevin. I mean, what do *you* like most?"

Kevin offered me another one of his dreadful, sugar-free cakes. "That I share my cookies."

*That's a damned good reason,* I thought. That's what all the great philosophers and religionists talk about. "Out of the mouths . . ." etcetera. But then the child startled me. No one had ever bothered to ask this before.

"What do you like most about yourself, Gary?"

I nibbled on the chocolate and thought of all my marvelous

attributes. I had such a selection, it was really difficult. He was looking at me with great interest, this enchanting, little boy. He was just one year younger than I was when I was first hit between the eyes with our disease. My countless virtues raced, in competition, to the tip of my tongue: my tolerance of stupidity, my great height, my patience, my even temper, my modesty. I could have gone on and on. Instead I told the truth.

"I try, Kevin. I try real hard. I never stop trying."